Outsmart
DIABETES

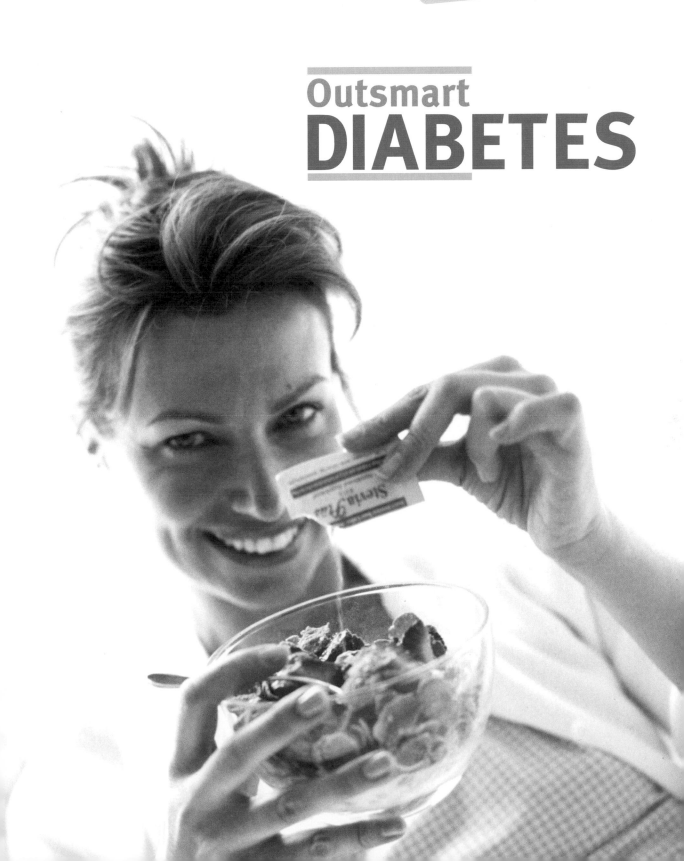

CONTENTS

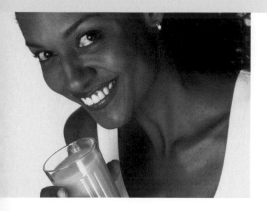

PART ONE: ABOUT DIABETES

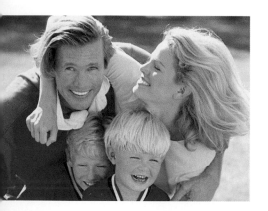

PART TWO: WHAT DOES DIABETES MEAN TO YOU?

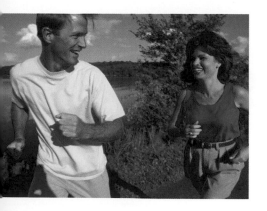

PART THREE: DIABETES AND YOUR FAMILY

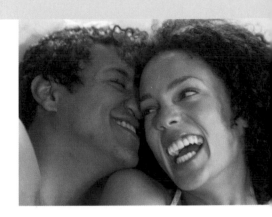

PART FOUR: CONTROLLING DIABETES

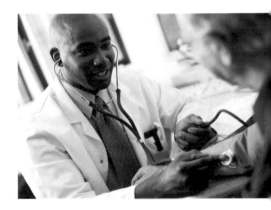

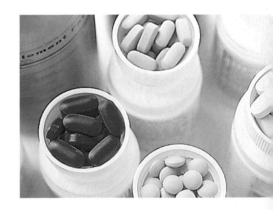

CONTENTS

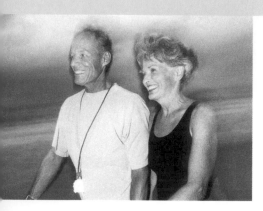

PART FIVE: GET FIGHTING FIT

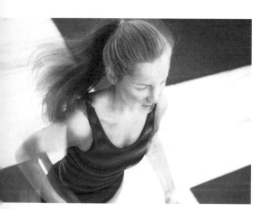

PART SIX: THE FOOD FACTOR

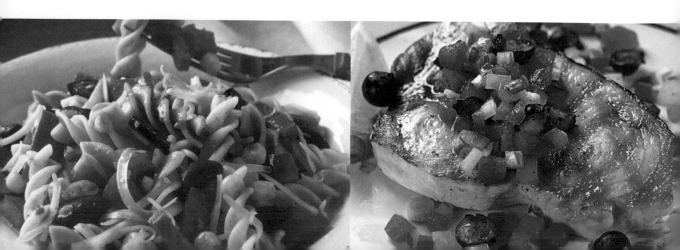

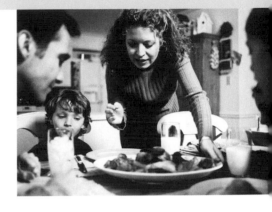

PART SEVEN: THE OUTSMART DIABETES COOKBOOK

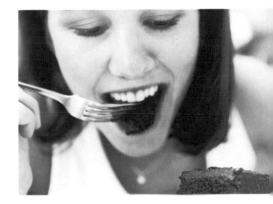

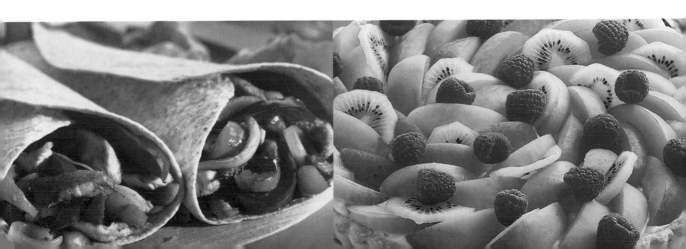

ABOUT THE PREVENTION HEALTH GUIDES

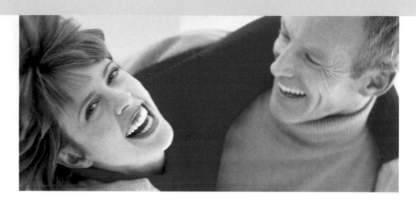

The Prevention Health Guides are a new and dynamic series of health books that are designed to fill the seemingly widening gap between the public's healthcare needs and the service available to them. The series' primary aim is to clear any mystery surrounding widespread ailments and put those suffering from them firmly in control of their lives, their futures and – as much as possible – their condition itself. The Guides achieve this by looking at all aspects of the illness and how to meet it head on, and recommend a series of all-embracing lifestyle changes that will raise your overall health and fitness levels to be at their best to outsmart your condition.

It should be remembered, however, that the Prevention Health Guides are not medical textbooks. They are not nearly that dry or exclusive. Prevention Health Guides are comprehensive, yet comprehensible explanations of common medical conditions. They are guide books in the true sense of the term, giving you instant health information on one level and providing a deeper, more theoretical understanding of the subject on another. They're like a traveller's guide book, offering instant access to a city in sharp soundbites and then a more thoughtful appreciation through detailed description.

The purpose of the Prevention Health Guides is to put you firmly in control. To enable you to talk to your doctor and other healthcare professionals with confidence and knowledge. To make you aware when you are getting less than first-class service and show you how to take charge if you still don't feel you are getting satisfaction. Prevention

Health Guides take an all-round approach to taking control, looking at every aspect of health, diet and fitness and how it can play a part in improving your life. So, in many cases this approach will offer a greater range of options than conventional medicine practitioners.

Prevention Health Guides are backed by *Prevention* magazine, the leading health and fitness magazine, which has a regular readership of over 12 million. This backing represents a vast range of expertise, resources and healthcare experience that provides the perfect foundation. From this unique perspective, Prevention Health Guides provide a new level of health and fitness advice for you and all your family.

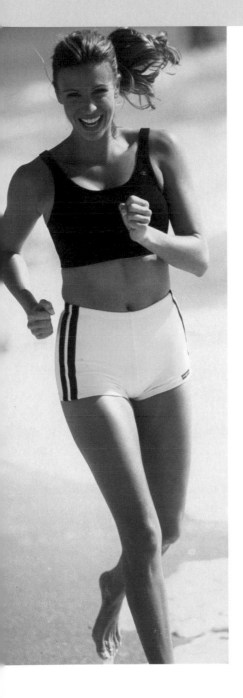

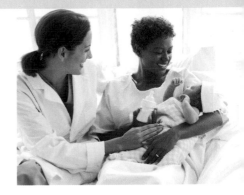

Everyone's heard of diabetes, but, like so many medical conditions, relatively few people know what causes it and how it's treated. So if you or a family member are diagnosed as diabetic, it can be terrifying – the first thing that comes to mind is a life of painful injections and never being able to eat chocolate again. *Outsmart Diabetes* has been put together to put right such misconceptions and to provide a whole range of information and advice, from recipes, exercise plans, conventional and holistic medicine through to methods for making school life easier for diabetic children. For the record, many diabetics control their condition through diet and exercise, and they can still eat chocolate.

We can't offer a cure for diabetes – no one can do that. What we can do is help you sort the facts from the fiction, so that you can feel confident about controlling your own health in partnership with your doctor and healthcare team. Learning all you can about your condition puts you at the centre of your own treatment.

Everyone is different, and once you've tried the recipes, and made time to exercise regularly, you'll find out what works best for you. Being diabetic means you become acutely aware of your diet and how your body feels as your lifestyle changes. With the right changes, the chances are you'll end up feeling better than ever!

The *Prevention* editors

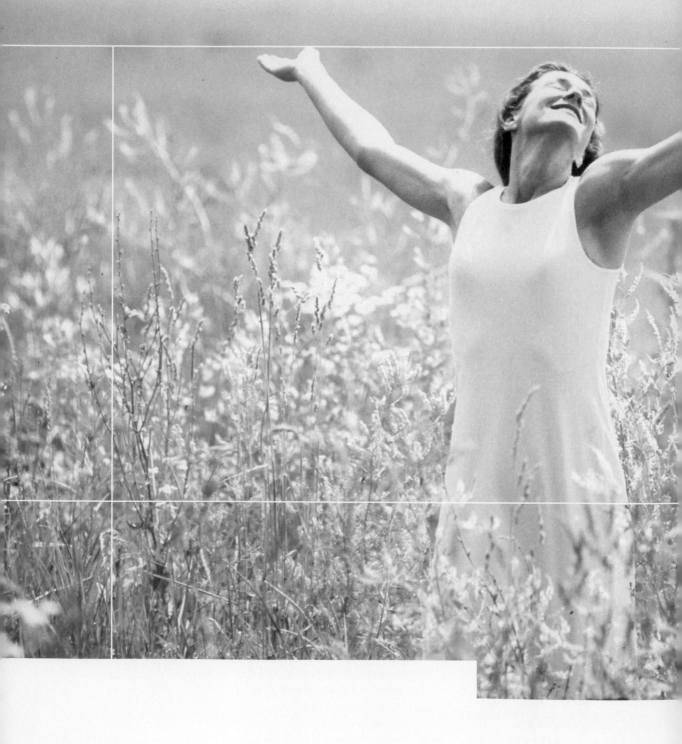

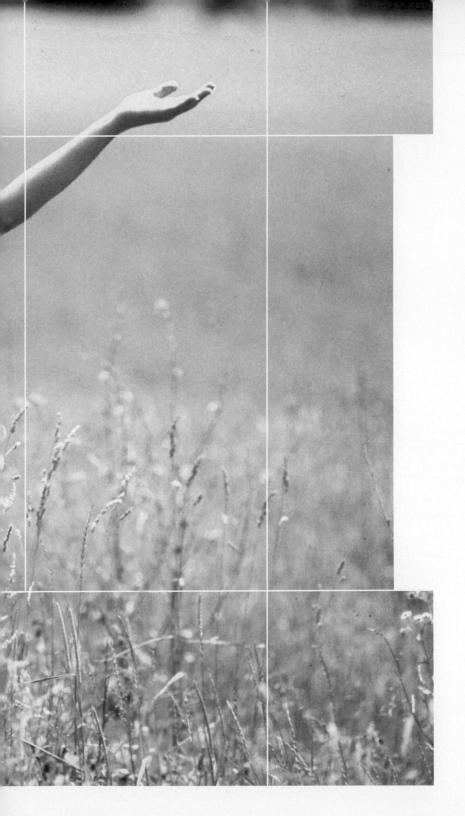

ABOUT DIABETES

WHAT IS DIABETES?

KNOWLEDGE IS EVERYTHING IN THE BATTLE AGAINST DIABETES. SO IF YOU'VE JUST BEEN DIAGNOSED WITH DIABETES, OR SIMPLY THINK THAT YOU MIGHT BE DIABETIC, IT'S IMPORTANT TO UNDERSTAND EXACTLY WHAT YOU ARE DEALING WITH.

THE TWO TYPES

TYPE I DIABETES

It is often referred to as juvenile-onset or insulin-dependent diabetes. Anybody, regardless of their age, sex, ethnic origin or weight, can have type I diabetes. The causes of type I diabetes are unknown, so it cannot be anticipated or prevented.

It means your pancreas doesn't produce any insulin.

You will have to give yourself regular insulin injections to compensate for the shortfall within your system as well as regulating your blood sugar. You will have to do this for the rest of your life.

TYPE II DIABETES

It is also known as adult-onset or non-insulin-dependent diabetes, this is most common in older and overweight people. However because our diet and lifestyle has changed so much over the past decades, becoming ever more unhealthy and sedentary, type II is developing with increasing frequency in young people, and seems to be linked to the growing obesity problem among adults (see page 66).

It means your pancreas makes insulin, but it either does-n't produce enough or your body isn't able to make use of it properly or efficiently.

You will have to lose weight if necessary, and adopt a healthy eating plan and exercise regime. But this may not be enough and your doctor may put you on glucose lowering pills and may even need to administer insulin.

DIABETES MAY BE IMPOSSIBLE TO CURE, but it can be controlled. And the first step in taking control of the condition is to understand it. In this case, knowledge is most definitely power. If you have been diagnosed as diabetic, it is important to realize you are not alone: diabetes is very common in the UK. There are approximately 1.4 million people who are known to have the condition, and up to another one million who have diabetes but don't yet know it. Of those that have diabetes, around 75 per cent have type II (see left).

First and foremost you have to be aware that when you have diabetes, something is wrong with the way your body produces insulin, a vital hormone made by your pancreas. When your body digests sugary or starchy food, it turns it into blood sugar, or glucose, in the liver and muscles, and uses this as fuel. Insulin helps your cells take in that fuel to power your muscles.

If you can't get glucose into your cells, they begin to weaken. Because your cells let your brain know they aren't getting enough fuel, your liver is triggered to pump even more glucose into your blood. After this, you'll start breaking down fat and protein as your body tries everything to get glucose into your body as usable energy. The sugar in your bloodstream builds up, potentially damaging everything from your organs to the blood vessels themselves. No wonder you feel tired, hungry and lose weight – no matter how

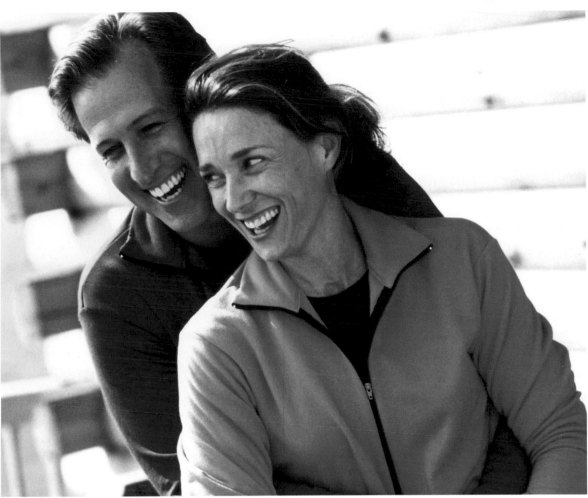

much energy you consume, your body can't make proper use of it.

Immediately beyond that though, you have to understand that not all diabetes is the same - there are two types, type I and type II, which are less commonly known as 'insulin-dependent diabetes' and 'non-insulin-dependent diabetes'.

If you have type I diabetes, your pancreas cannot create insulin. With type II, you can make insulin, but it is either not enough, or your body is not able to use it properly. Type I usually appears before the age of 40, and is treated by insulin injections, normally two or four times a day. Unfortunately, as yet insulin can't be taken orally because the digestive juices in your stomach would destroy it before it had a chance to work. Scientists are working on new treatments

for diabetes, but at the moment, if you have type I, you will have to have regular injections for the rest of your life. Type II diabetes is also sometimes known as 'adult-onset diabetes', because it occurs most often in people over 40. Sometimes, by carefully planning your diet and doing regular exercise, you can control type II diabetes without medication. But in some cases injections or tablets are also needed. Tablets work for type II diabetes but not type I because they don't contain insulin – they simply boost the effectiveness of the limited insulin that you produce.

Although they are two distinct conditions, in both types of diabetes the early warning signs are the same: feeling very thirsty, needing to go to the toilet all the time (especially during the night), unexplained weight loss, feeling ▶

JUST THE FACTS

DID YOU KNOW?
According to the World Health Organization, approximately 177 million people have diabetes worldwide, and this number is expected to reach 370 million by 2030.

Over 2 million people in the UK are known to have diabetes – that's about three to four in 100 people, but there is still an estimated one million others who are currently unaware that they have diabetes.

The number of people in Europe with diabetes is 32.2 million.

100,000 people are diagnosed with type II diabetes every day in the UK.

The term 'diabetes mellitus' comes from the Greek for 'fountain of sweetness', and derives from ancient physicians' observations that the urine of people with diabetes was sweet.

The peak age of onset in type II diabetes is between 60 and 70 years.

Currently, men are more likely to be diagnosed with diabetes because the only systematic screening for the condition in the UK is among the population with known coronary heart disease, which includes a much greater proportion of men.

The number of people in the UK who have type II diabetes but are unaware of it is estimated to be between 765,000 and one million.

In the UK, apart from natural causes, diabetes is in the top five leading causes of death, claiming more lives than AIDS.

The rate of lower limb amputation in people with diabetes is 15 times higher than in people without.

Diabetes is the leading cause of blindness among adults of working age.

Diabetes increases the risk of developing long-term complications such as heart and kidney disease, blindness and amputations. The condition also shortens life expectancy by up to 20 years for people with type I diabetes, and up to 10 years for those with type 2.

People with diabetes are entitled to free prescriptions and eye examinations under the NHS.

Diabetes accounts for around 5 per cent of the NHS budget at £3.5 billion a year – that's £399,543 an hour or £6,659 a minute.

Type II diabetes usually appears in people over the age of 40.

A key factor in the rise in type II diabetes is that, as a nation, we are increasingly overweight and less active.

Diabetes is up to six times more common among people of Afro-Caribbean and Asian origin living in the UK.

On average, if either parent has type 2 diabetes, the risk of developing the condition is 15 per cent. If both parents have type 2, the risk is 75 per cent.

Type I diabetes is more often diagnosed in children and young people, while type II mainly affects people over 40. However, more and more children are being diagnosed with type II.

In the UK, diabetes is the second most common cause of lower limb amputation because of ulceration.

People with diabetes must declare their condition when applying for motor insurance.

Movie stars Halle Berry, Sharon Stone and Elizabeth Taylor, all suffer from diabetes.

Five-time Olympic gold medallist Steve Redgrave was diagnosed with diabetes in 1997.

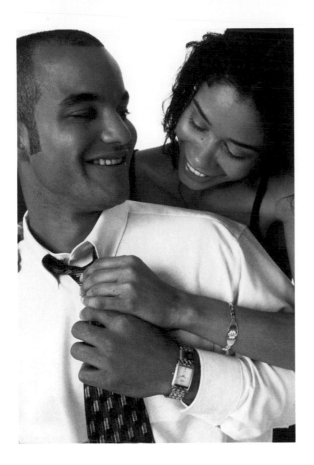

five times more likely to have the condition than their Caucasian counterparts. Of all type II sufferers in the UK, more than 80 per cent are overweight. Carrying extra weight makes you more likely to develop diabetes, and if you already have it, makes it more difficult to manage. That's why diet and exercise are essential to treating the condition. If you have high blood pressure, you are also at increased risk. Finally, diseases of the pancreas can also cause diabetes, though this is extremely rare.

As we've said, diabetes is a very common condition. And it can't be cured, but with the right combination of professional healthcare and a commitment from you, the individual, to choose a healthy lifestyle, it can be managed very successfully. Your next step is to follow our simple guidelines and take control. ◘

extremely tired or hungry, blurred vision, genital itching or regular episodes of thrush. If you suffer from one or two of these symptoms occasionally, it's easy to dismiss them as a result of a busy lifestyle, rather than a specific medical condition. This is especially true of type II diabetes, where the onset is slow. Many people have diabetes for years before they are diagnosed. But with the right treatment, the symptoms of both types can be relieved, and the sooner the condition is diagnosed, the less chance there is of any complications developing.

No-one is immune from developing diabetes, but there are some factors which put you at a higher risk. It runs in families, so if any of your relatives are diabetic you're in a higher-risk group right away. Type I is equally common in men and women, but type II is more common in women, because it can be connected with pregnancy (see page 47). Certain ethnic groups are also more likely to develop type II diabetes: people of Afro-Caribbean or South-east Asian origins are up to

WHAT IS KETOACIDOSIS?

If your body has had very high levels of blood glucose for a long time, it becomes overwhelmed by the sugar and begins to metabolize fat instead of sugar to provide energy. The breakdown of fat produces large quantities of ketones and acidosis, which makes the blood more acidic than the tissues of the body. When that happens you will get very ill. If the accumulation of acids and high blood glucose is very severe and the condition remains un-treated there is every chance you will fall into a coma. Most people with ketoacidosis are very dehydrated and will urinate frequently, they may also get an upset stomach that prevents them from keeping down any food. There is no way to anticipate ketoacidosis, and the best way to prevent it is to make sure you monitor your blood sugar and keep your levels under control. This condition is far more likely to occur in undiagnosed diabetics or those that aren't following a good health plan properly, as it requires a fair degree of neglect to take place.

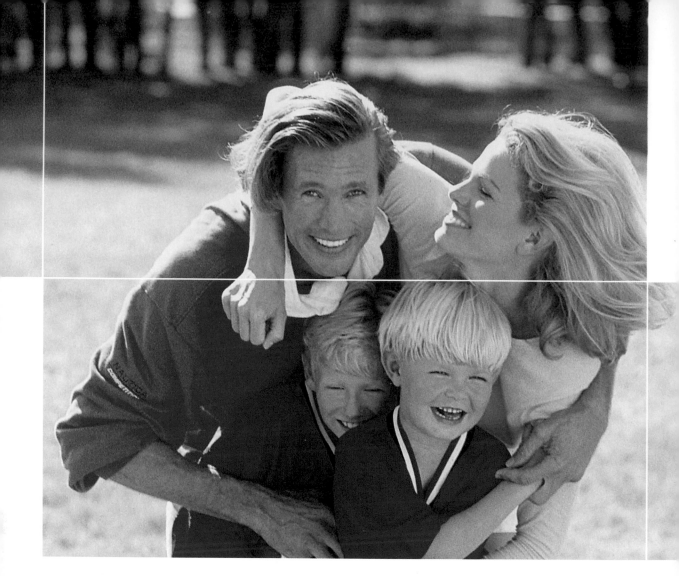

THE SIDE EFFECTS

IF YOU HAVE DIABETES, YOUR HEALTHCARE REGIME SHOULDN'T STOP AT THE CONDITION ITSELF. UNFORTUNATELY, UNCONTROLLED DIABETES CAN BRING ON A NUMBER OF RELATED CONDITIONS THAT YOU WILL HAVE TO GUARD AGAINST AS WELL.

BECAUSE DIABETES AFFECTS YOUR BLOOD sugar levels, it can reach every part of your body, from head to toe, via the bloodstream. Having diabetes means you have a higher risk of developing other health problems, including heart disease, stroke, high blood pressure and circulation problems. This in turn can lead to nerve damage, kidney damage and problems with your feet. There is also a risk of damage to your eyesight; one of the most common concerns of those diagnosed with diabetes is going blind. But don't panic. Blindness, kidney failure and heart disease are very serious complications, but they only arise if someone who is diabetic goes untreated, and does not manage their condition, for a very long time. With the right medication and the right diet and exercise routine, you and your healthcare team can eliminate almost all the side effects of diabetes, and any potential problems can be addressed as soon as they crop up. Early diagnosis and prompt treatment will keep you healthy and prevent any major complications before they arise.

Feet

High blood sugar levels can damage your nerve endings. This is called diabetic neuropathy, and results in an uncomfortable tingling, pain or numbness in the hands and feet, especially during the night. Combine this with possible circulatory problems and your feet are vulnerable. If you have lost some of the sensation in your feet, and the blood flow to them is restricted, any blisters, cuts or other small problems can escalate and become infected.

Around five per cent of diabetics in the UK develop ulcers on their feet every year. You can minimize the risk to your feet by always wearing roomy, comfortable shoes, and thick, soft socks. Check your feet regularly for calluses, cuts, bruises, and wash and dry them thoroughly, including between your toes. As romantic as it sounds, avoid walking barefoot on beaches and other outdoor places where there could be sharp stones, shells, rocks etc underfoot – if you can't feel your feet as well as you used to, you might not notice a small nick that could cause problems if left untreated. Foot spas may not be suitable for diabetics with neuropathy, so check with your healthcare team before using one.

If you have any problems with your feet, mention them to your doctor the next time you go for a check up. If your feet become suddenly swollen or discoloured, don't wait until your next scheduled appointment, it is vital to go and see your doctor immediately.

Skin

There is a vast network of capillaries carrying blood to and from the surface of your skin. When you have diabetes, these blood vessels can be affected, and in turn this can cause skin problems. Necrobiosis is a skin condition associated with diabetes that can be unsightly and painful. It is much more prevalent in female diabetics than males, but the risk of developing it is not altered by ethnic origin. Necrobiosis starts with small patches of skin becoming raised, almost like scar tissue, and it can be itchy or painful. Although it can make you feel self-conscious, it is not too serious unless the skin breaks, in which case there is a danger of ulceration or infection. Possible treatments ▶

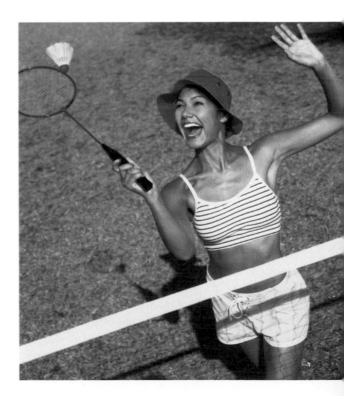

include UV light, or cortisone either as a cream or by injection, but there is no magic cure. Necrobiosis can happen to diabetics even if they keep their blood sugar levels within strict limits.

Kidneys

One in four of all diabetics will go on to develop nephropathy, or kidney disease. It is a slow process, and a sufferer may have had diabetes for 20 years or more before developing it. The best way to avoid it is simply to keep your blood sugar level between 4 and 8 mmol/l.

Your kidneys act as a filter, cleaning your blood and removing waste products into your urine. They also regulate salt levels in your system to control your blood pressure, and release certain hormones into your body. All of these functions can be impaired when kidney disease occurs. If you can't get rid of waste products from your blood effectively, they will build up in your body and make you extremely ill. If you are diabetic you should have your urine tested every year to monitor your kidney functioning, so that any problems can be caught as early as possible. If you do develop kidney disease you will have to control your blood pressure, and possibly modify your diet. In extreme cases, when your body cannot clean and filter your blood itself, dialysis may be the best option.

Heart

Diabetics are at least twice as likely as non-diabetics to develop heart disease, but, just like everybody else, there is plenty you can do to minimize your risk. First and foremost, quit smoking. Smoking just five cigarettes a day doubles your chance of heart disease, so don't just cut back, cut it out completely. Maintain a healthy weight, do regular exercise, let go of stress, and keep your cholesterol in check – all these common-sense health tips are even more important when you are diabetic.

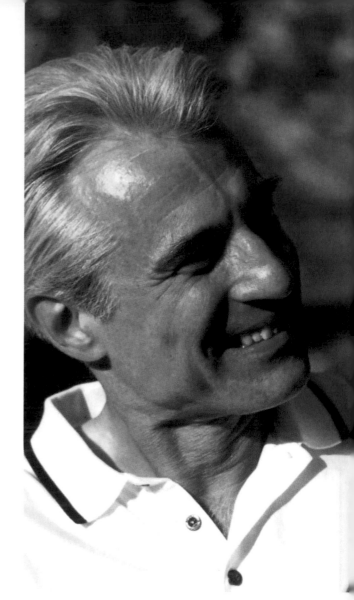

Stomach

As your body tries to cope with the effects of diabetes, it can play havoc with your digestion. Up to half of all type I diabetics suffer from gastroparesis, a condition that makes the stomach take too long to empty, although the majority of diabetics only have it mildly. Food travels through the intestines as it is digested, and that movement is controlled by a series of muscles that are in turn controlled by the vagus nerve. High blood sugar levels can damage this nerve and the blood vessels that supply it, inhibiting your body's ability to digest properly.

If food stays partially digested in your stomach for too long, it can form hard lumps (bezoars)

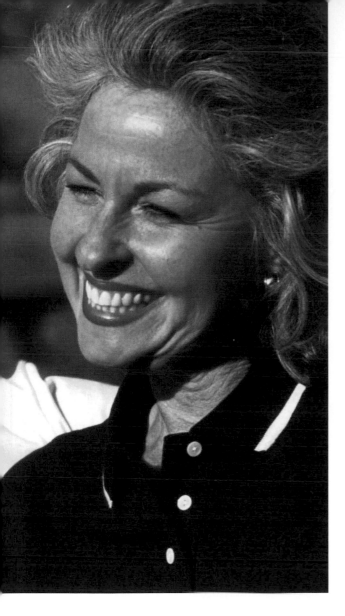

control can affect a woman's oestrogen levels, causing vaginal dryness and even urinary tract infections, while type II diabetes can also damage nerve endings. These side effects can make sex uncomfortable to the point of causing pain and are very likely to have a negative effect on a woman's enthusiasm for sex. However, dealt with promptly, these problems are treatable, and lubricants are widely available.

Although it's not true that diabetes causes impotence, there is a greater than average chance that diabetic men over the age of 50 will, at some point, experience difficulties in getting an erection. The secret is not to keep it a secret: talk to your partner and your doctor about what remedies may be appropriate. If you are having difficulty in this area, be careful not to drink too much and monitor your cholesterol level, as both can influence your ability to get and maintain an erection.

Osteoporosis

Osteoporosis, the debilitating loss of bone density, has been linked to both types of diabetes as a possible side effect. Studies have suggested that girls and young women with type I diabetes have lower bone density than their non-diabetic peers, considerably increasing their risk of bone fractures. While low insulin levels may be the cause, research is also examining levels of oestrogen linked to the bone-building hormone osteocalcin. Adult women with type I diabetes should have a bone scan at the first sign of menopause, and young or adolescent girls should make sure they get plenty of calcium.

In a US study of 10,000 women over the age of 65, those with type II diabetes were found to have an 80 to 90 per cent greater risk of hip and shoulder fractures than non-diabetics. However, research is, thus far, inconclusive as to why these figures are so high. ◻

that can block the small intestine. Alternatively, the undigested food can start to ferment inside you, causing nausea and vomiting. Of course these are symptoms of many conditions, or even food poisoning, so if you suffer from them, see your doctor to get a diagnosis. Gastroparesis is a chronic condition, so in most cases the best cause of action is to regulate blood sugar levels carefully and discuss with your doctor or healthcare team how to alter your diet.

Sexual health

Diabetes affects men's and women's sexual health differently, but none of the problems are incurable (see page 34). Poor blood sugar

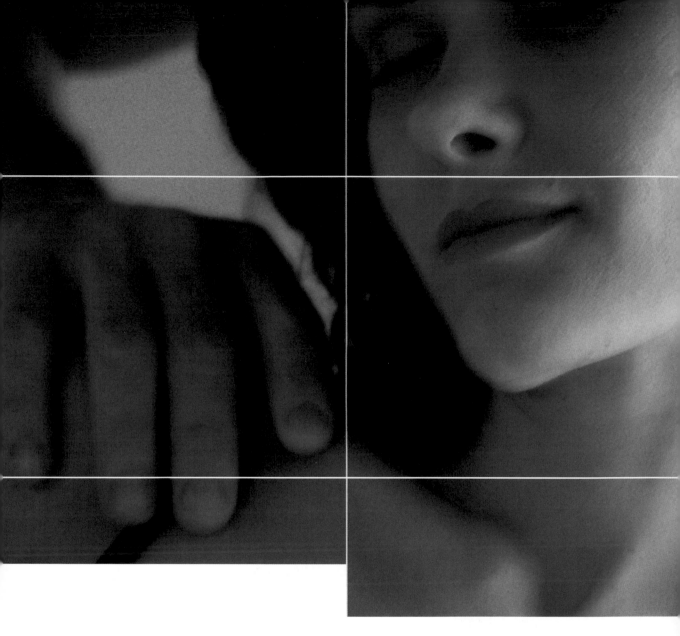

AM I DIABETIC?

TIRED? LOSING WEIGHT? ALWAYS NEEDING THE TOILET OR GETTING THIRSTY? IF YOU
THINK YOU MAY HAVE DIABETES, THE BEST THING TO DO IS FIND OUT FOR SURE.

YOU GOT A NEW PRESCRIPTION FOR YOUR
glasses six months ago, but you are having to
strain your eyes to focus on your computer screen
at work. It's been a while since you had a holiday,
and Monday mornings seem to come round
before the weekend is halfway through. You'd

probably feel much better after a couple of nights
uninterrupted sleep, but lately you keep having to
get up to go to the toilet.

Still, you've managed to lose a few of those
extra pounds without really trying – not bad for
someone who is the wrong side of 40. You decide

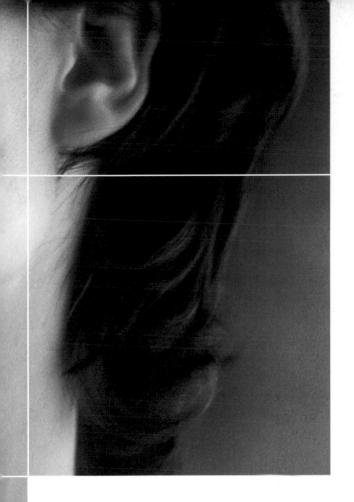

THE WARNING SIGNS

In type II diabetes, which typically develops in or after middle age, the signs may be very slow to manifest themselves, and are easily dismissed as an inevitable consequence of getting older, or simply not having enough hours in the day to do everything that you want. It is often only a routine medical examination that picks up the real reason. If you think you may be diabetic, keep a diary for a fortnight, looking out for all the symptoms listed below, then take the diary to your doctor and explain your concerns. These are the first signs that you may be diabetic:

- Increased thirst
- Needing to go to the toilet frequently, especially during the night
- Feeling extremely tired
- Feeling ravenously hungry
- Losing weight unexpectedly
- Blurry vision
- Genital itching or recurrent thrush
- Slow wound healing
- Dry or itchy skin

you just need a break from routine to refresh yourself in body and mind. In a typically busy life, it is easy to dismiss minor aliments and get on with the more pressing business of work, family, running a home and maintaining your social life. And usually, that's all those niggles are – minor ailments that can be fixed by a relaxing week away, with no stress, just lots of delicious, fresh food and a daily dip in the pool. But the problems don't always go away.

Many people are reluctant to go to their doctor, especially if they have a few different symptoms that, taken individually, don't seem worth mentioning. Who hasn't felt run down, or had a few days without managing to eat properly and then suddenly felt ravenously hungry and thirsty? And if they were individual symptoms, you might not be making a fuss. But as soon as they start adding up, it is vital that you start to take notice. Keep a diary of how you are feeling and what your key symptoms are over the course

of a week, and if you have several of the normal diabetes indicators, it is essential that you go and see your doctor. Tell him what you suspect you might have and make sure you include every aspect of your health and lifestyle.

If you so much as suspect you may have diabetes, the best thing that you can do is to find out for certain. That way, if you are diabetic, you can begin treatment promptly – by far the most effective way of dealing with the condition. If you are not, then you can eliminate any worries you have about being diabetic, and find out if there is anything else wrong with your health; you may simply be in need of a decent break. Diabetes UK (see p 156) estimates that one million people in the UK have diabetes, ▶

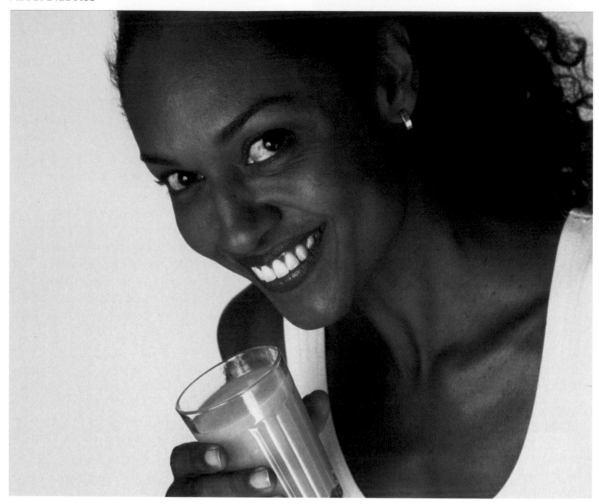

but haven't yet been officially diagnosed – make sure you're not one of them.

Stephen Nussey, a diabetes consultant at St George's Hospital in south London, says that getting an early diagnosis is absolutely essential. "The problem we have is that a lot of people don't realize that they've actually got diabetes." He suggests that anyone who has a close relative with diabetes, perhaps a parent or a sibling, should have a blood test once a year.

It is a simple procedure as just a few drops of blood are needed, and can be done at your doctor's surgery, or local hospital. It is best to have the blood test first thing in the morning, without having any breakfast, as you need to have had no food for 10 to 12 hours beforehand. Mr Nussey says it is a quick, simple test. "In the hospital we'll have the result that afternoon, and

your doctor will have it the next day."

Of all the symptoms that indicate a possible case of diabetes, Mr Nussey pinpoints thirst, weight loss (he suggests a drop of 3–4 kg/6.5–9 lbs without any change in diet) and needing to dash to the toilet all the time as the most significant. He says that "Three or four litres of urine a day, rather than the normal two" is the amount an undiagnosed, untreated diabetic is likely to pass.

So if you even suspect you might be at risk of having diabetes, make an appointment with your doctor straight away. A quick, painless blood test will tell you if you are diabetic. Knowing the facts is more than half the battle, so make sure you're not one of the million people who are suffering in silence. Once you have a positive diagnosis, you can plan your treatment programme, and get on with the rest of your life. ◘

WHO'S AT RISK?

There is no way of knowing who will develop type I or type II diabetes – anyone could, but some people are more susceptible than others. These are the factors that put you at a greater risk of becoming diabetic:

AGE
Type II diabetes is the most common form of the disease, and, as its former name adult- or maturity-onset diabetes implies, it usually occurs among the over-40s. The older you get, the greater your risk of developing this form of diabetes.

DIABETES IN THE FAMILY
Diabetes isn't passed down directly from parent to child, but if someone in your family is diabetic, then you are at a slightly increased risk. The closer the relative, or the more diabetic relatives you have, the greater the risk – if both your parents are diabetic the risk is raised considerably (see The Probability Panel, page 46).

ETHNIC ORIGIN
People of Afro-Caribbean or South-east Asian origin are three to five times more likely to be diabetic than Caucasians. Recent studies have shown that over 20 per cent of Indian men over the age of 50 are diabetic.

WEIGHT
Some 80 per cent of the million people in the UK with type II diabetes are overweight. The more overweight you are, the greater your risk of diabetes, not to mention heart disease, high blood pressure and other health problems.

DIABETES AND PREGNANCY
When you are pregnant, you can develop gestational diabetes (see pages 47) that lasts for the duration of your pregnancy. Having gestational diabetes means you are more at risk of developing type II diabetes in later life, and more likely to give birth to a big baby weighing more than 4 kg (9 lb).

HIGH BLOOD PRESSURE
Having high blood pressure doesn't cause diabetes, but if you do have high blood pressure, you are automatically putting yourself in a higher risk group for diabetes. And if you have diabetes already, having high blood pressure makes it worse, and can accelerate complications. It makes sense to keep your blood pressure under control, whether or not you are diabetic.

SEDENTARY LIFESTYLE
If you have a sedentary job, and don't take regular exercise, you are increasing your risk of developing diabetes. You're more likely to be carrying extra weight as well, and this is another risk factor.

HIGH CHOLESTEROL
Having elevated cholesterol levels is bad for your health in all sorts of ways — it increases your risk of heart disease and stroke, as well as diabetes.

PANCREATIC PROBLEMS
If you have have suffered damage to your pancreas – often brought on by long-term alcohol abuse – or you have had an operation on it, your beta cells may be damaged or you may not be producing enough digestive acids to break your food down properly. And either of these conditions can affect blood sugar.

STEROIDS
The higher the amount of steroids you're taking, the greater your chance of becoming diabetic. The greater the amount of steroids, the greater the boost to your blood sugar. However, they create a dependency that means that, even if you stop taking them, you will remain diabetic.

SELF-ASSESSMENT QUIZ

THE EARLY SIGNS OF DIABETES CAN BE EASY TO MISS. THAT'S WHY
WE'VE PREPARED THIS SIMPLE, SELF-ASSESSMENT TEST.

Q1. How often do you sleep right through the night?
(a) Always, unless my daughter is having a sleepover and there are giggles coming from her room all night.
(b) I occasionally have to get up to get a glass of water or use the toilet.
(c) I rarely sleep through until morning without having to go to the toilet.

Q2. What's the first thing you do when you wake up?
(a) Check that the children are up and getting ready for school.
(b) Put the kettle on and open the post.
(c) Run straight to get a glass of water or straight to the toilet.

Q3. How do you feel after a lie-in on a Sunday morning?
(a) I don't like to lie in past eight o'clock. There's so much I want to be doing with the kids on a weekend, it seems like a waste of time.
(b) An extra hour in bed is wonderful because it makes me feel refreshed for the rest of the day.
(c) I'm so exhausted that lying-in until lunchtime still leaves me feeling sleep-deprived.

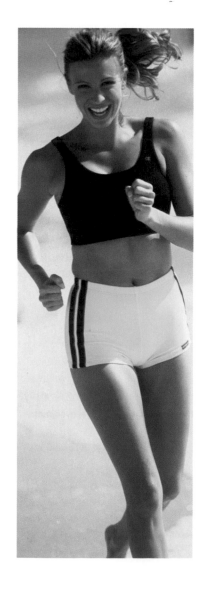

Q4. How well have you maintained your weight in the last month or two?
(a) I've been making a real effort to eat better, and it's starting to pay off – I've steadily lost weight.
(b) It's stayed about the same.
(c) Actually, I seem to have lost weight without changing my diet.

Q5. How good is your eyesight?
(a) I need glasses for reading, but other than that it's fine.
(b) I've worn contact lenses for years, so I go for regular check-ups and there are no problems.
(c) I got new lenses for my glasses six months ago, but I'm already finding it difficult to read the text on my computer screen. I think I may need a new prescription.

Q6. If you have children, how much did they weigh when they were born?
(a) Mine are twins, so they were only 2.2 kg (5 lb) each.
(b) My first was 2.7 kg (6 lb), and my second 3 kg (7 lb).
(c) I've only had one baby so far, and he was a bouncing 4 kg (9 lb) when he came along.

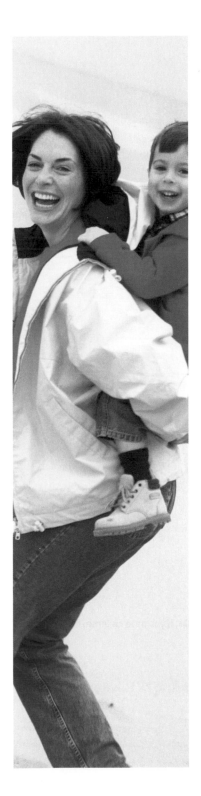

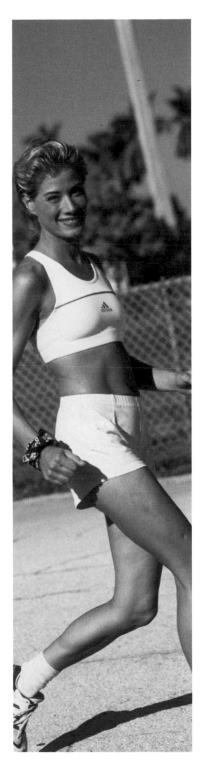

Q7. If you nick your finger, how quickly does the wound heal?
(a) Within a few days.
(b) Pretty quickly, but I always use some antiseptic cream just in case.
(c) Sometimes it takes ages to clear up completely, even if it's a minor cut.

Q8. Generally speaking, how good is your skin condition?
(a) I've got a few laughter lines, but that's because I laugh so much.
(b) My sister took me for a facial for my birthday, so I'm feeling radiant.
(c) It seems to be getting much drier, but maybe that is just me getting older.

If you answered 'c' to three or more of the questions, you have at least some of the characteristic signs of diabetes. If you are overweight, or have a family history of the disease, it is even more likely that you have developed diabetes. Of course filling in this quiz is designed to make you think about your health, it's not a way of doing a medical diagnosis. However slight your suspicions, if you think you might be diabetic, go and see your doctor and ask for a blood test.

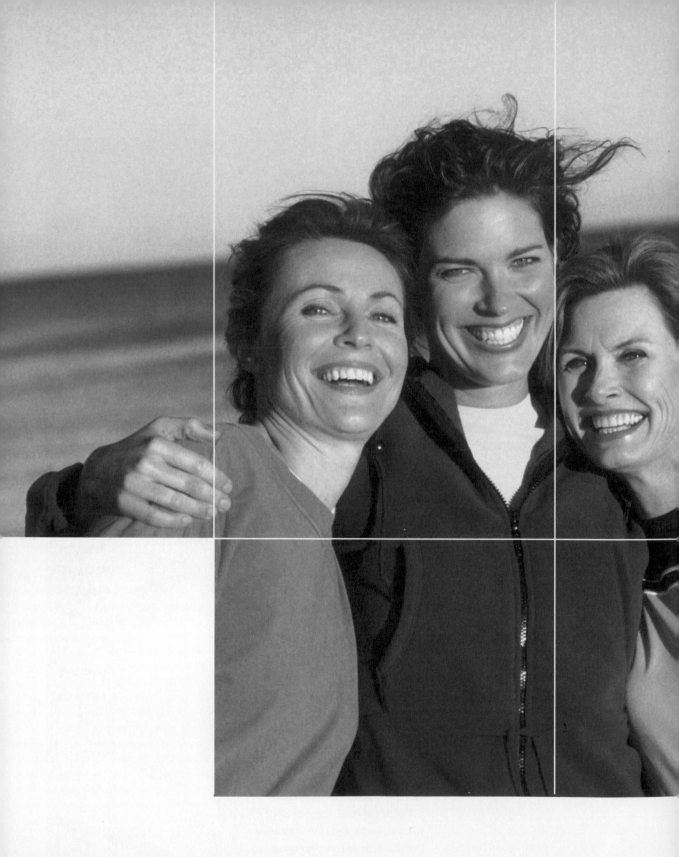

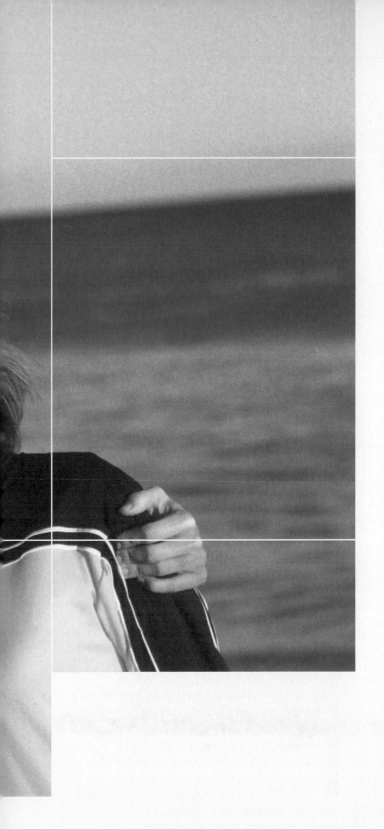

WHAT DOES DIABETES MEAN TO YOU?

YOU'VE JUST BEEN
DIAGNOSED

IT MAY COME AS A SHOCK, BUT BEING DIAGNOSED WITH DIABETES ISN'T THE END OF THE WORLD. WITH A FEW, SIMPLE LIFESTYLE CHANGES YOU MAY EVEN END UP FITTER AND HEALTHIER THAN EVER.

WHEN YOU SIT DOWN WITH YOUR doctor and are told that you are diabetic, you're going to need some time to take it in. The chances are you'll be out of the surgery door and halfway home before your mind starts brimming over with all the questions you should have asked while you were in the consulting room, but of course you were too overwhelmed to think of them on the spot. Saying 'don't panic' is easy. Not panicking can be tough, especially if all you know about diabetes is that it means injecting yourself every day for the rest of your life, risking going blind and never being able to eat chocolate again – none of which need be true. The best way to dispel your fears is to learn about your condition, and take control of it.

For many people, a diagnosis is actually a relief. It explains the perpetual thirst, feeling run down, unexpected weight loss and all the other unexplained symptoms that have been disrupting your life. The chances are you'll be happier and healthier as a well-informed diabetic than you were as an undiagnosed one.

And if your family make some of the lifestyle changes with you – so you eat well at meal-times, and make time to exercise together – they'll get to be in better shape too. Being diabetic means you'll learn about how your body really works, and how you can get the most out of it.

As a diabetic, you will develop a relationship with your doctor that you haven't previously had. You'll go for regular check-ups, and as you get to know each other you'll find communication easier. But you won't be handing control of your health to your doctor – you have to remain at the centre of your own treatment. Aside from the lifestyle changes you make, the most obvious example of this is that you will have to test your own blood sugar. Almost all blood sugar meters work by pricking your finger and taking a drop of blood. The amount of blood is very small, so it doesn't hurt. Just remember to test on a different finger each time. If you keep using the same one it will get sore. It's important to keep a good record of your blood sugar level, and look out for any highs or lows. Doing this will give you greater control of your condition, because although you may not feel any different, if your blood sugar keeps creeping up you're increasing your risk of developing complications.

If you have type II diabetes, you may be able to control your condition with diet and exercise, and possibly oral medication. Some type II diabetics, and all type Is, will need to inject insulin. You have to inject it because if ▶

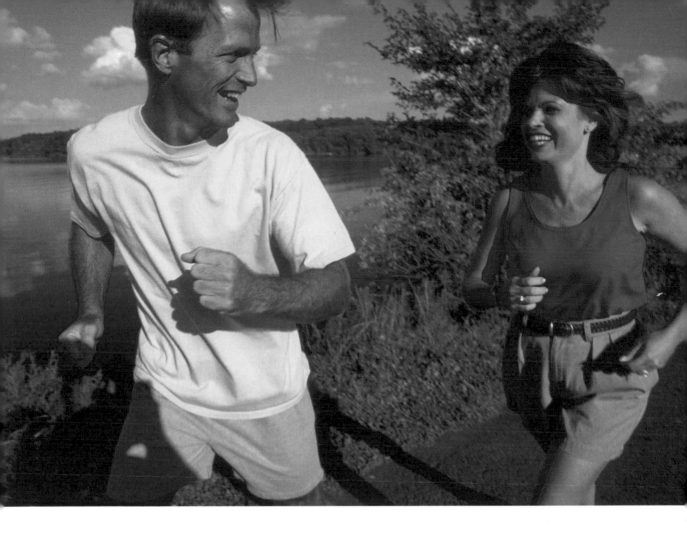

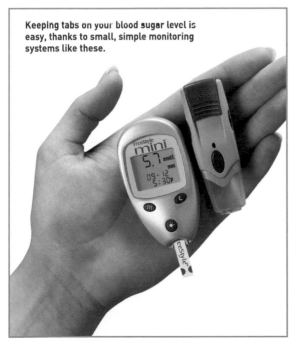

Keeping tabs on your blood sugar level is easy, thanks to small, simple monitoring systems like these.

HOW DO I TEST MY BLOOD?

As a diabetic, you will have to carefully monitor and record your blood sugar levels, by supplying a small amount to a specialist blood sugar meter for instant analysis. There are many meters on the market, and all are straightforward to use, discreet and small enough to be easily transported. They vary from hi-tech models that keep records for you and mark trends in your readings, to basic and functional versions that merely indicate your blood sugar level at the time of the test. But the good news is that the amount of blood they need to draw is now very small indeed, which is just as well, as you're going to have to get used to using the monitor regularly. The key to controlling diabetes is self-management. Constant monitoring and recording of your blood glucose levels is vital if you're to stay on top of your treatment.

you took it as medicine your digestive system would break it down before it had a chance to get to work. Scientists are working on other ways of taking it – for example as an inhaler, similar to those used by asthmatics – but for now, injecting is the only way. You'll have to inject two or four times a day, so however daunting it seems at first, you'll soon get used to it. Diabetes UK (see page 156) estimate that 700,000 people in the UK inject insulin every day. Your doctor will explain the process to you and help you learn how to do it. There are different sorts of insulin. Some work almost immediately and need to be injected just before or after a meal. Others types are slow-release, which you inject once a day, usually in the evening. It's up to you and your healthcare team to decide what is best for you.

Traditionally, diabetics take insulin using a syringe. Nowadays these are disposable, so there's no risk of infection from repeated use. If this is what you opt for, your doctor will provide you with information about the safe storage and disposal of needles. Many people prefer to use an insulin pen – it's more discreet, and with disposable cartridges, isn't messy either. Whichever method you use, most needles are not very long, and are very fine. To get used to injecting, it might help to put an ice cube on the injection site for a few moments beforehand to numb it slightly. You need to inject subcutaneously (into the fat under your

THE DIABETIC'S DICTIONARY

One of the most unnerving aspects of being diagnosed as a diabetic is the amount of baffling medical jargon that comes your way. It is almost impossible to take control of your situation if you can't communicate with your doctor, other healthcare workers or even fully understand what you are reading. Here's a list of some terms you are most likely to come across as you strive to find out more about your condition.

ARCABOSE
A drug that blocks the digestion process that turns sugar into glucose

ACIDOSIS
A higher than normal acid level in the bloodstream

ATHEROSCLEROSIS
Clogging up and eventual hardening of the arteries

BACKGROUND RETINOPATHY
The type of retinopathy (disease of the eye) most common to diabetics

BLOOD GLUCOSE OR BLOOD SUGAR
The level of glucose/sugar in the bloodstream

BLOOD PRESSURE
The pressure at which blood is pumped through your arteries

CARBOHYDRATES (OR CARBS)
Starchy or sugary food, producing simple sugars – glucose – when digested

CARDIAC (OR CARDIO)
Of the heart

CELLS
The basic material, as very small units, that make up the human body

CHIROPODIST
A foot specialist

CHOLESTEROL
An animal fat that gets into the bloodstream, and comes mostly from meat, dairy and poultry

DIABETES MELLITUS
A condition where the glucose levels in the bloodstream are too high

DIABETIC AMYOTROPHY
Usually called neuropathy, this is the nerve damage attributed to diabetes, which causes wasting of the muscles

FIBRE
Indigestible bulk in food that aids digestion and can help control blood glucose levels

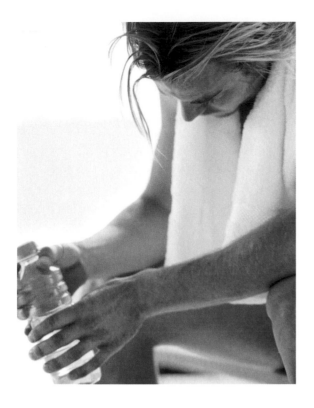

skin), not into a muscle or blood vessel. The easiest places to do this are the thighs, buttocks and tummy. If you don't have much body fat, pinch your skin and inject into the fold, rather than straight into your flesh. And try to inject into different sites, rather than the same place all the time.

An alternative way to take insulin on board is via a pump. This is a device about the size of a deck of cards, with a thin tube that attaches to a needle that goes under your skin, providing a continuous flow of insulin. If you want to use an insulin pump you will need a good understanding of how your eating patterns, insulin and blood sugar work, and have to monitor your blood sugar very carefully. ◘

GLUCOSE
Carbohydrates are metabolized into this simple sugar that circulates in your bloodstream to provide energy

GLYCOGEN
Glucose stored in the muscles

HYPER
Too high: hyperglycaemic – high blood glucose levels; hypertension – high blood pressure

HYPO
Too low: hypoglycaemic – low blood glucose levels; hypotension – low blood pressure

INSULIN
This hormone produced in the pancreas is the catalyst that carries glucose from the bloodstream into the cells to provide energy

INSULIN-DEPENDENT DIABETES
Type I diabetes, occurs when the body doesn't produce enough insulin

JUVENILE-ONSET DIABETES
Type I or insulin-dependent diabetes, as it occurs in children and young adults

LIPID
The overall term for fats as they occur in the human body

METABOLISM
The process of breaking down foods in the body

MONOSATURATED FATS
The most healthy of the 'good' fats, found in olive oil and groundnut oil

NON-INSULIN-DEPENDENT DIABETES
Type II diabetes, which is due to the body not being able to use its insulin properly, rather than not having enough. Does not normally require insulin dosage.

OBESE
Very overweight

POLYUNSATURATED FATS
'Good' fat, found in fish oils, olive oil and soya beans

PROTEIN
The nutrient – found in high quantities in meat, poultry, fish and dairy – that is needed for cell growth and repair

SATURATED FATS
'Bad' fats, found in meat and dairy products

THROMBOSIS
Blood clotting

TRIGLYCERIDES
Fats that are found floating in the bloodstream

TYPE I DIABETES
Insulin-dependent diabetes

TYPE II DIABETES
Non-insulin-dependent diabetes, that can usually be managed by diet and lifestyle changes, instead of injecting insulin

JUST BEEN
DIAGNOSED FAQs

WHENEVER YOU FACE A NEW CHALLENGE THERE ARE ALWAYS LOTS OF QUESTIONS. BEING DIAGNOSED WITH DIABETES IS NO DIFFERENT, SO HERE'S A QUICK RUN-THROUGH OF SOME OF THE MOST COMMON CONCERNS.

Can I eat foods with sugar in them?
Yes. As part of a balanced diet, diabetics can have occasional sweets or chocolates just like anyone else. If you take insulin, or certain tablets to control your blood sugar, you may sometimes even need to eat high-sugar foods to stop your blood sugar from dropping too low.

What's a 'hypo'?
Hypo is short for hypoglycaemia, which mean low blood sugar, below 4 mmol/l. Hypos usually happen when you have too much insulin in your system, or not enough food, but sometimes there is no obvious reason for them. If you have a hypo you will feel dizzy and hungry, you will be pale, and unable to think straight. Your vision might start to blur, or your lips tingle. As soon as you feel any of these symptoms starting you must get some sugar into our system, either glucose tablets, sweets or a fizzy drink.

Will I pass on diabetes to my children?
Not necessarily. Type II diabetes can be inherited so if there is a history of it in your family then it does put your children in a higher risk group, but if they keep active, eat a balanced diet and maintain a healthy weight, they will be less likely to develop the condition.

Am I going to lose my eyesight?
No. If you follow your healthcare team's advice, eat sensibly, take your medication as prescribed and control your blood sugar levels, and don't smoke, your eyesight will not be affected by your diabetes. But you should go for eye tests, or fundo-scopies once a year, and if you do notice any blurring in your vision, tell your doctor immediately.

Will I have to inject insulin for the rest of my life?
If you have type I diabetes then yes, you will have to inject insulin for the rest of your life. If you have type II, however, it depends on your exact medical state — it may be enough to maintain a healthy diet and lifestyle, or you made need to take tablets. Only some type II diabetics need to inject insulin.

Can diabetes be cured?
No, not yet. Scientists are developing and refining treatments for diabetes all the time, so that it is easier to manage, and there is also ongoing research into a cure or even a vaccination. Currently scientists are working on a vaccine that has had success at immunizing mice from diabetes, but it will be several years at least before they will have developed a safe human version of the drug.

Will I be able to donate blood?
If you are on any type of medication, be it injections or tablets, then no, you won't be able to donate blood. However, if you are a type II diabetic, control your condition by diet alone and are otherwise healthy, the National Blood Service would welcome you as a potential donor. You will be asked to attend a session where a doctor will assess your suitability as a donor. Contact the National Blood Service (see page 156) to find the location of your nearest session.

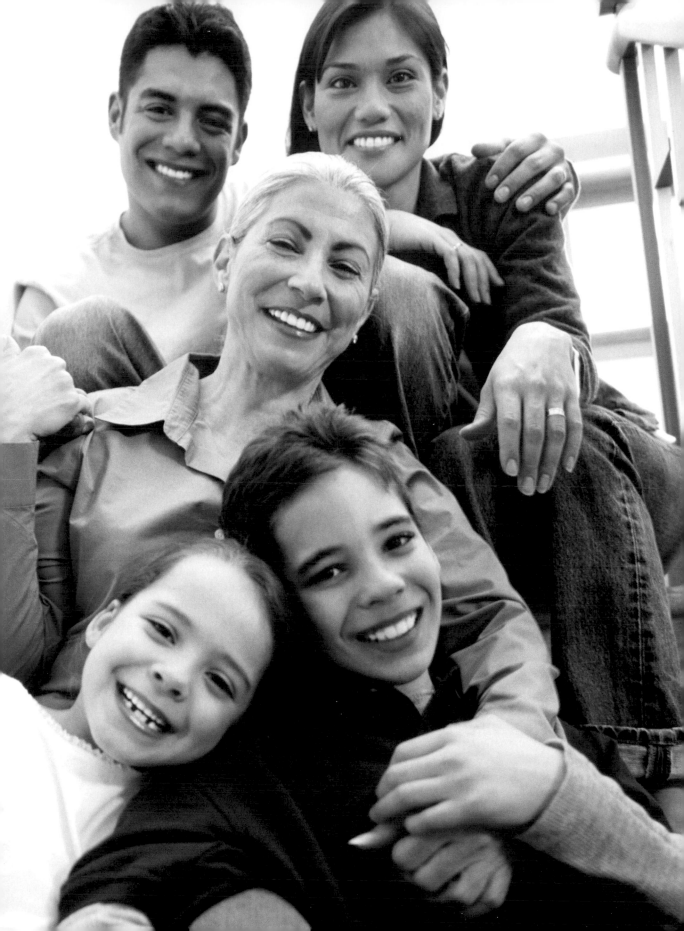

SEX AND THE SUGAR

DIABETES NEEDN'T DAMPEN YOUR LOVE LIFE, BUT HEALTH PROBLEMS OR THE WORRIES RELATED TO DIABETES CAN HAVE AN EFFECT IN THE BEDROOM. BUT YOU DON'T HAVE TO SAY GOODBYE TO YOUR SEXUALITY, JUST TAKE STEPS TO KEEP YOUR ARDOUR IN AS TIP-TOP CONDITION AS THE REST OF YOUR BODY.

FACE UP TO IT TOGETHER

For men and women with diabetes who find themselves facing these problems, the most important thing is to talk to your partner about what's going on in your body. If your partner is helping you take control of your diabetes, there is no reason why he or she will not be sympathetic to this unfortunate side effect. Make lovemaking a priority. Sex is part of a normal, healthy lifestyle, and there's no reason for diabetes to stop that.

MAKE SURE YOU TALK TO YOUR DOCTOR

Don't wait for your doctor to bring up the subject of sexual difficulties, as the chances are he or she won't – even if they have been treating your diabetes for years. A recent survey found that 63 per cent of diabetes patients – both men and women – who had experienced sexual difficulties as a side effect had never been asked about any such possibilities by their doctor.

IF YOU OR YOUR PARTNER SUFFER FROM diabetes, being able to communicate and support one another is more important than ever. But it isn't always easy, especially since diabetes can have knock-on effects in the bedroom. It affects men and women differently, but it's important to remember that none of the problems are incurable. Correct management of blood sugar will make an enormous difference.

Undiagnosed diabetes often leads to loss of libido in both men and women, but this is more about being ill than being diabetic. When anybody is under the weather, for practically any reason, their sex drive is one of the first things to be affected. And because diabetes is a serious condition, affecting your energy levels and your entire body, it is no surprise that the libido often suffers. The good news, though, is that this is not strictly a diabetes-related problem. And so once you have realized what you are suffering from –

and have taken the appropriate steps to get control of – it, your sex drive should gradually return to normal.

For women, poor blood sugar control can cause some more serious problems. If badly mismanaged, it can affect oestrogen levels causing vaginal dryness, and in more severe cases chronic yeast and urinary tract infections. This can make sex uncomfortable or downright painful. Further affecting a woman's enthusiasm for sex is the possibility that type II diabetes can lead to damaged nerve endings, also causing discomfort. Taking control of your blood sugar levels is the best way to combat the cause of these problems, while any dryness can be overcome by the use of lubricants. These can be bought over the counter at chemists, but if you use condoms choose a water-based lubricant, as oil-based ones can damage the latex and trigger infections. If you feel you need oestrogen medication you will have

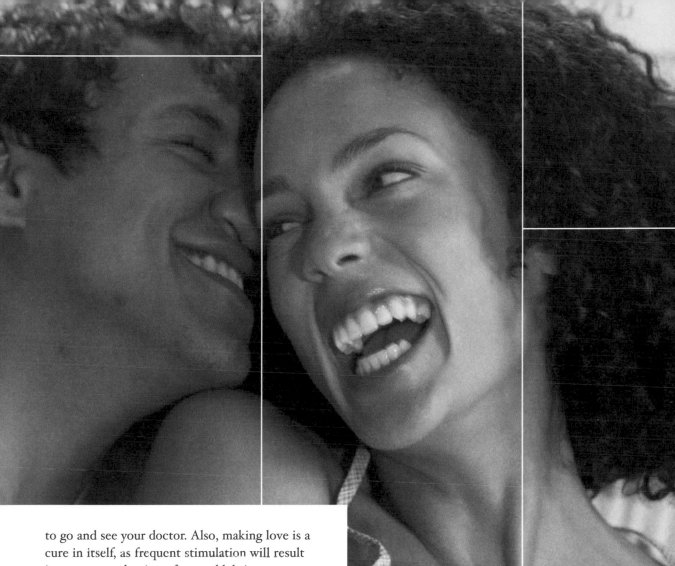

to go and see your doctor. Also, making love is a cure in itself, as frequent stimulation will result in greater production of natural lubricants during intercourse.

Diabetic men aged over 50 have a 50-60 per cent chance of having trouble getting an erection. Nerve and blood vessel damage is usually to blame because diabetes will have an effect on blood flow to the extremities. But as is often the case with non-diabetics too, the problem is just as likely to be psychological. And we certainly shouldn't forget that diabetics frequently worry about their condition and, if they're not fully in control, will be physically far from 100 per cent healthy, a factor that can also prompt erectile dysfunction.

If you're too hurt and embarrassed to admit you have an erectile problem, focus on the underlying cause. Failed erections are almost always a symptom of something else – in this case, diabetes. Talk to your doctor about your difficulties, and discuss the range of treatments available to find one that suits you. Also make sure you take control of the situation yourself by making sure you are in optimum health and thus minimizing any extraneous problems. Drinking too much alcohol can lead to similar problems for non-diabetics, but it will be more acute for a diabetic. Too much cholesterol in your blood can make matters worse too, and lack of exercise and a bad diet will remove your drive and add to any general feeling of malaise. Finally, certain medications, including antidepressants, cardiac medicines and antihypertensives, often prescribed for diabetes-related complaints, can cause impotence as a side effect. ◘

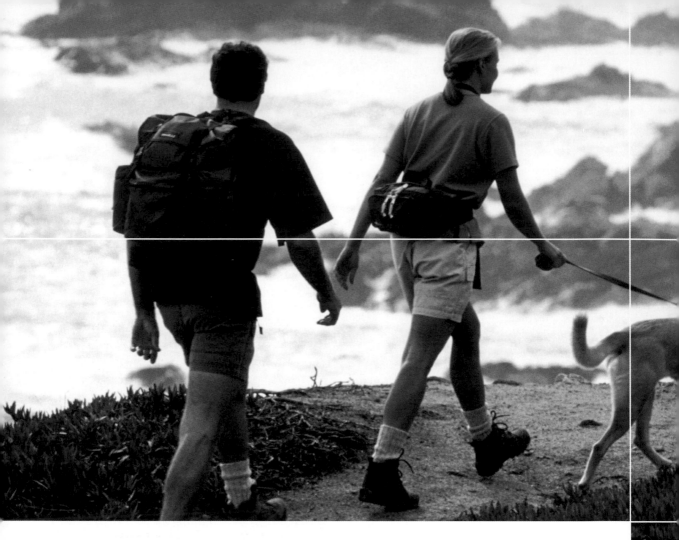

ENJOYING TRAVEL

FOR A NEWLY-DIAGNOSED DIABETIC, LIFE DOESN'T CHANGE THAT RADICALLY, SO
THERE'S NO REASON WHY YOU SHOULDN'T CONTINUE TO ENJOY FOREIGN TRAVEL.
JUST MAKE SURE YOU STAY FIRMLY IN CONTROL OF YOUR CONDITION.

MONEY, PASSPORT, TICKETS, SUNTAN lotion, phrase book... getting ready to go on a family holiday can be a stressful experience, and if one of you is diabetic, there are even more things to think about. What will you be able to eat? Can you take needles on board a plane? What if you have a hypo in the hotel bar?

Away from home, with its familiar foods, a friendly doctor at the end of the phone and a network of supportive friends, you need to take special care to control your diabetes. With common sense and planning, you and your family will be able to enjoy a well-deserved break without compromising your treatment.

Since 11 September 2001, airlines, have been understandably more security conscious than ever. Sharp instruments – scissors, penknives etc – must not be carried in hand-baggage. But of course type I diabetics will almost certainly have to carry syringes or an insulin pen with them during their

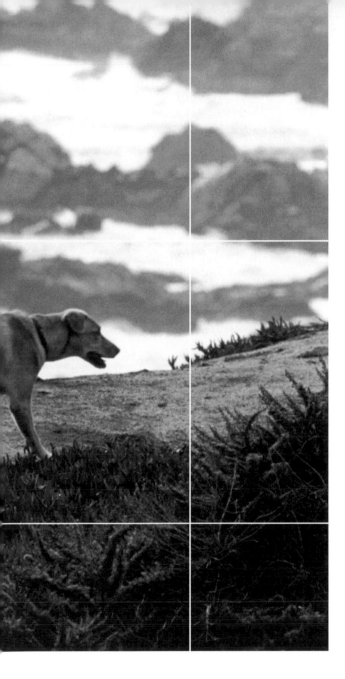

BEFORE YOU GO

Once you have booked your holiday, there are certain essential preparations for every diabetic about to travel:

■ Visit your doctor for advice and a letter explaining your condition
■ Inform the travel company or agent you have booked with that you are a diabetic
■ Contact the airline to get their advice on flying with syringes in your luggage – American airports and airlines are particularly strict
■ Also, make sure the airline knows you are a diabetic and inform them of any dietary requirements
■ Stock up on medical supplies. Take twice the amount you think you would need at home. This applies to everything: insulin; syringes; needles; glucose-lowering tablets; glucose tablets; blood testing equipment; urine testing strips; and so on. You will need to give your doctor and pharmacist advance warning that you are going to require such a large amount at one time
■ Make sure you have plenty of any specialist footcare products
■ Contact the hotel or wherever you are staying to make them aware of your condition
■ If you are going to a hot country and don't have a fridge in your room, organize portable storage for insulin to keep it at the correct temperature (4-25°C/39.2-77°F)

flight. If you did put insulin in the hold it would be damaged by the very low temperatures, so even if you don't think you'll need to inject during the journey, you should keep your insulin with you. Get a letter from your doctor before you go, certifying that you are diabetic, and explaining your needs. If you are a frequent traveller, ask for a letter that you can use each time you fly. Tell the airline staff when you check in that you are diabetic. They may ask you to hand your medication to a steward during

the flight, and only ask for it back if you need to inject, you should carry it in a separate bag that you can give in if required.

Part of the fun of visiting new places is enjoying a different lifestyle, and trying new foods. Providing you stick to a broadly healthy diet, there is no reason why you can't sample local delicacies, but be sensible – don't eat food that has been out on a roadside stall all day, no matter how colourful and tempting it looks. An upset ▶

DON'T LEAVE HOME WITHOUT ...

When you are abroad and out and about visiting historic sites, shopping or just lounging on the beach, there is an essential diabetic's travel pack you should put together, stow in a bag and carry with you at all times. These are items over and above your medication, and it forms a kit that, especially if you are going around by yourself, will ensure your holiday is as risk-free as possible, so you can enjoy your trip without too much worry. And above all, don't forget to replace any of the food and drink items as soon as they are used.

■ Your diabetic identification, whether it's a medallion or a bracelet
■ Your diabetic card

■ A letter from your doctor explaining your diabetes and its treatment, and any allergies or relevant peculiarities
■ A letter in the languages of the countries you are visiting explaining you are a diabetic and what to do in an emergency
■ A list of emergency phrases in the languages of the countries you are visiting – it may help you to print these out phonetically as well
■ A mobile phone that is operational wherever you are going; or a cache of local coinage to allow you to use public telephones
■ Bottled water
■ A glucose drink
■ A high-carbohydrate energy bar

stomach can spoil anyone's holiday, but if you are diabetic it will play havoc with your blood sugar levels. If you do suffer, drink plenty of bottled water or diet soft drinks, and take glucose tablets to get some energy into your system. Make sure you check your blood sugar every couple of hours – you may well need to boost the amount of insulin you are taking while you are ill.

Whether you are seeking sun and relaxation or snow and winter sports when you leave Britain, you're going to be in a different climate, and that can affect some aspects of your diabetic self-care. If you suffer from neuropathy (see page 17), particularly in your feet and lower legs, make sure you have appropriate footwear. Wearing sandals will expose delicate skin to the sun, so make sure you don't burn the tops of your feet. If your feet are prone to problems, you may be best to stick to wearing trainers: sand and grit can easily get into sandals and cause irritations that you might not notice immediately. Going barefoot also puts you at risk of treading on broken glass, cigarette

ends or sharp shells, so if in doubt, keep flip-flops on in the sea, and wear cotton espadrilles to keep the sun off your feet.

In cold climates it's more important than ever to keep your circulation pumping. If you are hiring ski-boots, explain that you are diabetic and take extra care when being fitted.

If you are going somewhere exotic, and need to take malaria tablets, or have immunizations before you go, talk to your doctor and get them done in plenty of time. If you are going somewhere where you don't speak the language, commit a few useful phrases to memory so that you can at least tell people that you are diabetic and that you take insulin. If you are worried about pronunciation, write the phrases down and carry them with your other documentation.

Wherever and however you travel, it's important that the people around you know you are diabetic. Make sure you inform your holiday company, airline, hotel reception or bed and breakfast owner, and if they haven't had experience of

IN THE AIR

Once you have informed an airline that you are diabetic, make sure you have more than enough medication for the duration of the flight and that it is stored correctly. Regardless of what conversation you may have had at check-in regarding your diabetes, talk to the cabin crew once you are on board to make sure they are aware of the situation. Monitor your blood sugar more frequently than usual, as the stress involved in flying, the irregular meals and unusual food can have an effect. Rather than attempt to adjust your medication timetable as you pass over different time zones, it will be much more convenient for you to continue as if you'd never left home, and only change your schedule to your destination time zone when you actually touch down. There is nothing inherently wrong with this, but once again, it will require particularly vigilant monitoring of your levels, especially if you have a long drive after a long flight.

a diabetic customer before, explain what it means. Always carry plenty of food and bottled or canned drinks with you – shops may shut at lunchtime, or during religious festivals – and a good first-aid kit. It should include all the necessary diabetes medication you would normally use in a day, and all your testing equipment: finger pricker, blood-testing strips, urine-testing strips, glucagon, glucose tablets and a letter from your doctor.

Insulin has to be stored at between 4–25° C (39.2-77° F), so it will need to be in a cool bag. And don't forget that if you are travelling across time zones you will have to adjust your insulin routine. Keep checking your blood glucose level and have regular snacks. It might be easiest to keep your watch set to UK time until you arrive, and not adjust it back until you are home. If you are properly prepared, you won't come back from your holiday in need of another one. ◘

LOOK AFTER YOUR FEET

As a diabetic, foot care will already be high on your list of priorities, but once you get on holiday your feet will be particularly vulnerable. Heat, long walks, sand, dust, sharp rock on the sea bed and going barefoot all conspire to increase your risk of foot infection. Talk to your doctor and your chiropodist before you set off, and make sure

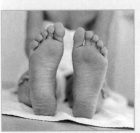

you follow any specialist advice they might give you, then follow these simple guidelines:

■ Never wear new shoes when on holiday, especially if the weather is hot
■ Take comfortable, well-fitting shoes
■ Don't wear sandals as it leaves your feet in danger of being cut or nicked and you're likely to accumulate dust between the leather and the tender skin on your feet
■ Especially avoid wearing flip-flops as the unforgiving plastic bar between the toes can easily chafe and result in an open sore
■ Don't go barefoot on the roads or footpaths
■ Be extra vigilant as to what is on the seabed
■ If you have no access to a washing machine – and rinsing out in the hotel room sink doesn't count! – take far more clean socks than you think you will need
■ Wash your feet thoroughly more than once a day, and don't put dirty socks back on clean feet
■ Always wear clean shoe liners in your trainers

Diabetes UK (www.diabetes.org.uk) can provide a wealth of vital information for the diabetic. They also provide invaluable support for people with both type I and type II diabetes, as well as their family and carers.

DIABETES
MYTH BUSTIN'

DIABETES TREATMENT HAS CHANGED A LOT OVER THE YEARS, AND AS UNDERSTANDING OF THE CONDITION HAS INCREASED, MANY OF THE 'RULES' HAVE BEEN SET ASIDE. BUT THAT DOESN'T STOP THEM REAPPEARING FROM TIME TO TIME, SO HERE'S A LOOK AT THE REAL STORY BEHIND TEN OF THE MOST FREQUENTLY CITED DIABETES MYTHS.

THERE ARE A LOT OF 'TRUTHS' TOLD about diabetes, diabetics and what they can and can't do – and most of these concern what they can't do. While some of these pieces of wisdom might have been fact a few years ago, when much less was known about diabetes and its treatment, now understanding and taking control of diabetes is such that many of these old adages no longer stand up. As a newly diagnosed – or even veteran – diabetic it's very important that you don't scare yourself or restrict your lifestyle by confusing fact with fiction.

YOU CAN'T HAVE SUGAR

You can if you're careful. Sugar is a fast-acting carbohydrate that, if eaten by itself, such as in a fizzy drink or sweet tea, can push your blood sugar levels dangerously high. But if you limit your intake, eat it as part of a larger, balanced meal and adjust your medications and your intake of other carbohydrates to compensate, there's no reason why you can enjoy the odd cake (see The Outsmart Diabetes Cookbook, page 121).

YOU CAN'T DRINK ALCOHOL

Once again, moderation is the key. Alcohol can impair the liver's response to low blood glucose levels, but that will only happen if you drink large amounts. Also, be aware of the amount of sugar in alcohol as part of your carb-conscious eating plan.

YOU WILL HAVE TO PLAN YOUR LIFE AROUND YOUR INJECTIONS

Not necessarily. Insulin pens are a far more discreet and portable way of taking insulin. Then there is the increasingly popular insulin pump that delivers insulin gradually throughout the day, allowing you to remain in full control of your situation.

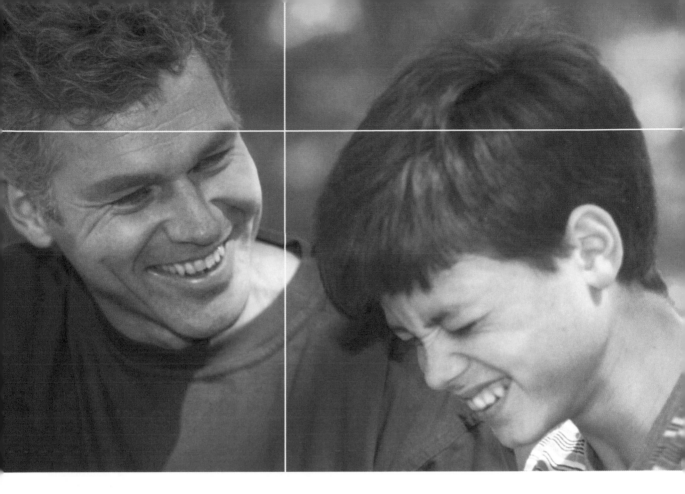

YOU CAN'T HAVE KIDS

Of course you can, but you will need to be very careful to correctly manage your blood sugar levels and to follow a strict healthy eating plan before conception, during the pregnancy and while breastfeeding.

DIABETES IS CURABLE

No, unfortunately it isn't. This is the one negative point as regards these most popular diabetes myths, but with a careful eating and exercise regime you can take control of it to such a degree that it is entirely manageable.

YOU WILL BECOME IMPOTENT

Impotence affects most men at some time in their lives and the causes of it are legion. As a healthy diabetic you are no more susceptible to it than non-diabetics. But the stress is on the word healthy, as impotence is frequently caused by nerve and blood vessel problems, which can be a diabetes side effect. On the plus side, though, as erections rely on healthy blood flow and your eating plan is designed to give you exactly that, you could actually be protecting yourself against becoming impotent.

YOU ARE DIABETIC SO YOUR CHILDREN WILL BE, TOO

There is a considerably higher chance they will be if both parents are non-insulin dependent diabetics, but it is still far from a foregone conclusion.

YOU CAN'T PLAY SPORTS AGAIN

Of course you can. Carefully monitor and maintain your blood sugar levels before, during and after competing, and take on the required extra carbs. Also be sure your teammates understand your condition.

YOU CAN'T EAT OUT

This is not true. Merely apply the same rules to eating out as you would to eating at home (see page 115) – cut back on what's bad for you and and enjoy what's good for you.

YOU CAN'T GO ON HOLIDAY

You can (see pages 36-9). Just make sure you have diabetic indentification on your person at all times, follow the airline's regulations for carrying syringes on a flight and learn 'I'm a diabetic' in the language of wherever you are going.

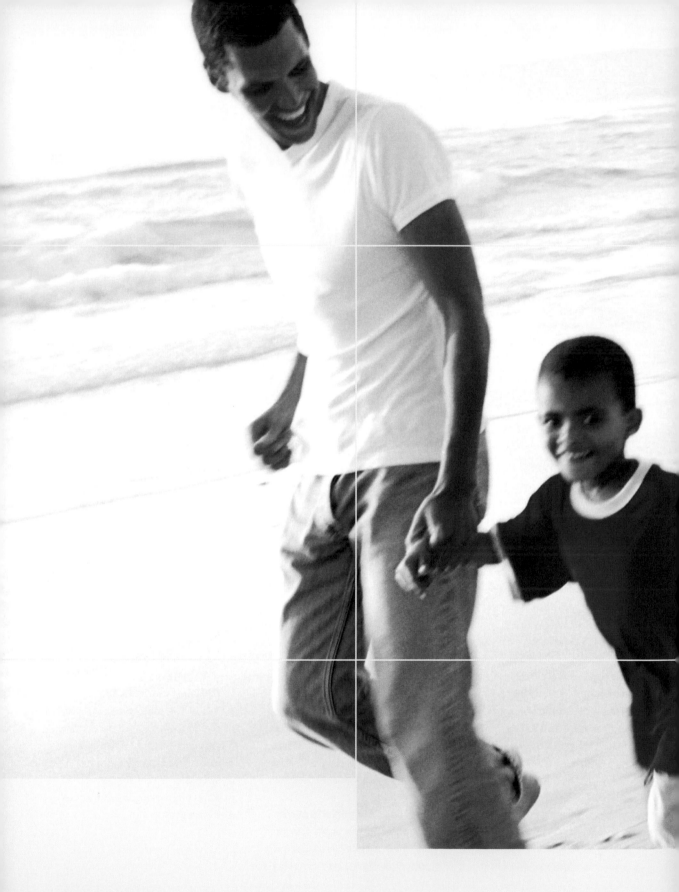

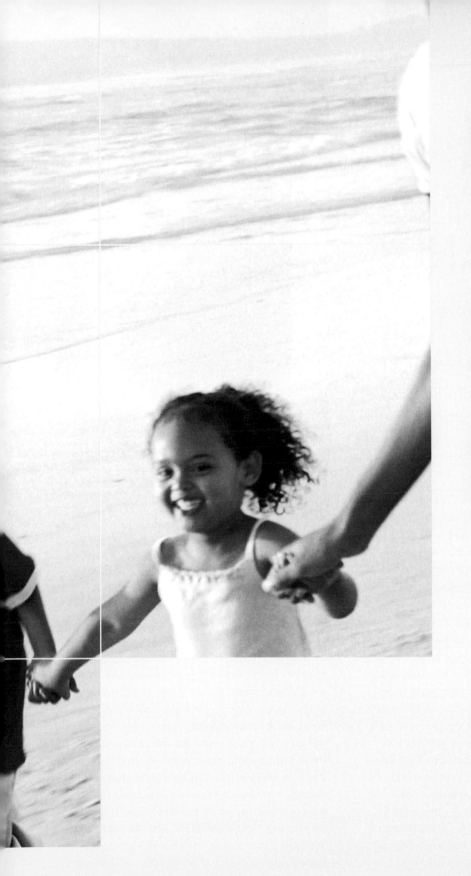

DIABETES AND YOUR FAMILY

ENJOY A HEALTHY PREGNANCY

FOR A DIABETIC WOMAN TO ENJOY A HEALTHY PREGNANCY, SHE'LL HAVE TO WORK HARDER TO STAY IN CONTROL OF THE CHANGES TO HER BODY. BUT THE REWARDS SHOULD BE WORTH IT!

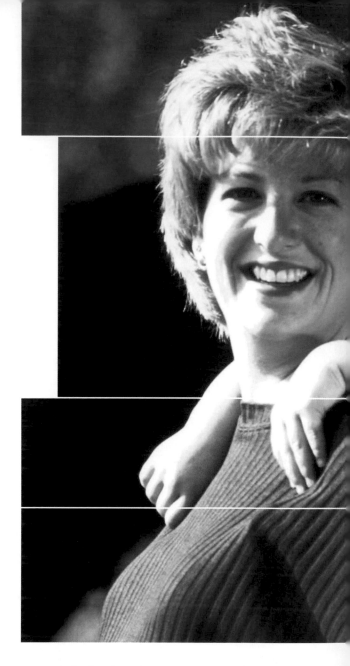

IF, AS A DIABETIC, YOU ARE PLANNING a pregnancy either to start a family or add to an existing one, you will need to talk to your doctor. At this very early stage your doctor will advise you on how best to approach conception from a health and a psychological standpoint. The latter is a big part of these discussions; to be as relaxed as you should be about this stage in your life, you'll need to be aware of the facts relating to a diabetic's pregnancy. Remember, you can't stay in control unless you have all the information.

It is equally important that your partner be involved with these discussions too. While you should already have talked as a couple, at length, about actually having a baby, your partner will have to be aware of any complications that could arise. Because you'll increasingly come to rely on him, he has to feel able to ask questions and feel very involved at this stage.

Once you've got past the initial questions and have decided to go ahead, the real work begins! All sorts of strange things happen to every woman's body when she is pregnant, and if you are diabetic these changes need to be managed to the tiniest detail – even prior to conception. Being in optimum health while trying to conceive will give you a head start on the extra strength you'll need for the months ahead. In this respect it is now more important than ever that you manage your blood glucose levels as closely as possible, because you'll need to maintain optimum energy levels and make sure the inevitable hormone fluctuations don't do you any harm. Statistically, the greater proportion of diabetic

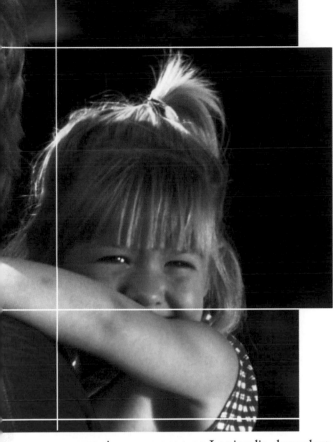

DAD'S BOX

Too often fathers complain that they are all but ignored during a pregnancy – that their work is done – but as a diabetic you cannot afford to leave your partner out of the equation. As your pregnancy progresses, you are going to need far more support, both emotionally and physically, than a non-diabetic. In fact you and your baby will be happier, healthier and, above all, safer if you let dad take his share of the strain, so make sure he:

■ Is able to recognize the symptoms of hypoglycaemia, especially at night, as that is when hypos commonly occur during pregnancy. Uneven breathing and a lot of movement are the obvious symptoms.
■ Knows where there is a supply of glucose (including glucagon) and can administer it in an emergency under stressful conditions.
■ Has learned how to administer insulin in whatever form you take it.
■ Can take your blood sugar readings for you
■ Is as involved as possible with visits to the clinics and takes part in the discussions with your doctor to fully understand how your condition affects your pregnancy.
■ Creates as stress-free an environment as possible for you in order for your pregnancy to be a relaxed and happy one.

GET YOUR EYES TESTED

As a diabetic, you are already more vulnerable to eye problems arising from swellings in the capillaries (aneurysms) due to increased blood flow. When you become pregnant there is a very good chance your blood pressure will rise and so considerably raise this risk. It is crucial, therefore, that you get a thorough eye examination to allow your optician to detect any signs of damage as early as possible.

pregnancies are among type I or insulin-dependent diabetics, simply because they tend to be younger than type II diabetics who are unlikely to have developed the disease before they reach their 40s. If you are an insulin-dependent diabetic and take oral medication, your doctor will probably switch you to injecting during pregnancy. Even as a non-diabetic, there is a chance you may develop gestational diabetes, a specific form of the disease which only occurs in pregnancy. Although it needs to be carefully managed with diet and physical activity, there is a large probability it will disappear after you have given birth.

Once you become pregnant you must stay in regular contact with your doctor, as your condition can potentially increase the risk of several diabetic complications: retinopathy, high blood pressure, kidney disease or neuropathy. But while these are only possibilities – they ▶

THE PROBABILITY PANEL

If you and/or your partner has diabetes, what are the chances of your children being diabetic? Taking parentage as the sole contributor, the probabilities are:

■ If both parents have insulin-dependent diabetes (IDDM), the chances are 35 per cent

■ If the father-only has IDDM the, chances of his child developing it are 10 per cent

■ If the mother-only has IDDM, the chances of her child developing it are 2 per cent

■ If neither parent has IDDM but they already have a child that has, the chances of their next child developing it are 8 per cent

■ If both parents have non-insulin dependent diabetes (NIDDM), the chances of their child developing it are 75 per cent

■ If either the mother or the father has NIDDM, the chances of their child developing it are 20 per cent

■ If the mother develops gestational diabetes, even if it does not remain, the chances of the child becoming a diabetic are slightly higher than otherwise.

These figures are not scientifically accurate, and are changing constantly as the incidences of diabetes increase across the board.

BACK HOME

Once you get your baby home, don't neglect your diet as it is particularly important you maintain your healthy eating plan. If you are breastfeeding, you may have to increase your carbohydrate intake, so make sure you compensate for that in other areas. Be careful not to allow yourself to become dehydrated by paying particular attention to how much water you are drinking. And try not to put on extra weight, which is easily done if your sleeping and eating patterns are thrown out by the baby's demands and you find yourself eating snacks at odd times of the day and night.

are possibilities that will decrease in relation to how healthy you stay – one thing your doctor will immediately do is adjust your insulin levels. Your requirements will increase and he will carefully monitor this in response to your blood sugar readings – by the end of your term you will probably need twice as much as your pre-pregnancy dosage. Understandably, one single injection a day might not be able to deliver your daily needs correctly, so you may have to perform more than one jab a day or even switch to an insulin pump.

One of the reasons for the dramatic rise in insulin requirements when you are pregnant, is because of the actions of the placenta. Your placenta will act as a channel for your baby, passing nutrition and oxygen in one direction, and expelling waste products in the other. On the downside, it also produces several hormones, some of which can inhibit the effectiveness of insulin. As your pregnancy progresses and the placenta grows, it will produce more of these hormones and your pancreas will try and compensate by generating more insulin, but it won't always be able to keep up with this renewed demand. While this will be expected and accommodated for in diabetics, it is this condition in non-diabetic pregnant women that leads to gestational diabetes.

In most cases, gestational diabetes can be controlled by diet, but in about a third of cases, you'll need to inject insulin. Although it is usual for gestational diabetes to disappear after the birth, it can put you at a higher risk of developing type II diabetes so your doctor will ask you to come in for tests after you have had your baby to check that everything has returned to normal.

Throughout your pregnancy you will have to monitor all aspects of your condition, from checking your blood glucose levels at least four times a day through to eye tests every three months and, importantly, your calorific intake. It is tempting to think that eating for two can become an excuse for overindulging, but you'll need to be very careful of weight gain outside that which is normal in a healthy pregnancy. Don't forget, the extra weight will bring with it all the dangers associated with obesity and diabetes in non-pregnant women. At the beginning of your pregnancy, you should not eat extra calories – instead, you should simply stick to a healthy eating plan. You should only eat about 200 extra calories more a day when you reach their third trimester (from 28 to 40 weeks). Be very aware that the more excess weight you carry, the more insulin you will need, and the more strain you will be putting on your cardio-vascular system in general.

While the risk of having a hypo is greater when you are pregnant, there is no evidence that hypoglycaemia will harm your unborn baby. However, it is very important that those around you – family, friends, colleagues and so on

– know how to recognize the symptoms of a hypo and how to treat it by administering sugary food or drinks, or, in extreme cases, by giving you a glucagon injection. Make sure you keep drinks or snacks to hand at home, at work or with you when you are out, as well as wearing or carrying some form of diabetic identification. Should you allow your blood sugar to get totally out of control you could suffer from ketoacidosis (see page 15), which in the most extreme cases can be fatal. It occurs when your blood sugar gets extremely high – often if you have some sort of infection – and causes all the symptoms you'd expect: extreme thirst, hunger, confusion and weakness. You can check if you're at risk by using ketone testing strips – this is a simple urine test, much like the one you did to see if you were pregnant – then if there is anything untoward you can go straight to your doctor for treatment if necessary. ▶

GESTATIONAL DIABETES

If you develop gestational diabetes, and between 2 and 5 per cent of expectant mothers will, it just means you'll have to be more careful about your health. Try not to worry – with proper treatment it can be easily controlled.

HAVE I GOT IT?

Because gestational diabetes is relatively common, women should be screened with an oral glucose-tolerance test between 24 and 25 weeks of pregnancy. While it's vital you don't miss this test, you can have it earlier in your pregnancy to put your mind at rest.

WHY HAVE I GOT IT?

The placenta can produce a hormone that blocks the efficient usage of insulin in your bloodstream, thus extra supplies have to be taken either by injection or a pump.

WILL MY BABY GET IT?

By the time gestational diabetes is detected, a baby's organs are already fully formed so it won't develop diabetes. The only real problem might be that babies of mothers with any form of diabetes tend to be larger, which can result in early labour being induced or a Caesarean section.

WILL IT GO AWAY?

Gestational diabetes usually disappears after the birth as your body returns to normal. However, make sure you are tested for type II diabetes at your postnatal check ups, because diabetes is one of its risk factors.

WILL IT HAPPEN AGAIN?

If you have had gestational diabetes already, it is far more likely to occur in future pregnancies.

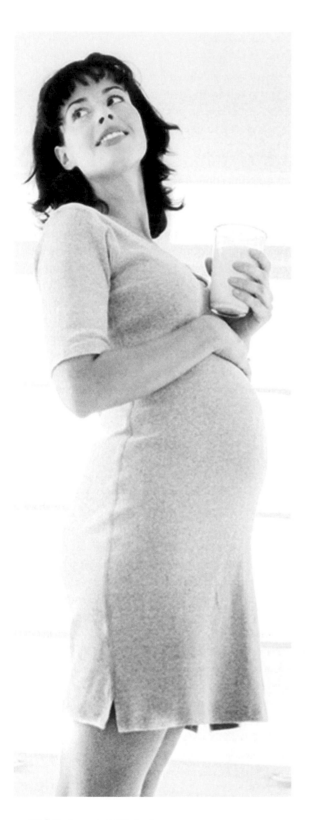

At the birth, whether you have type I, type II or gestational diabetes, you are likely to have a big baby, as your raised blood glucose levels will have meant he or she will have been getting extra fuel for growth while in the womb. The technical term for this is 'macrosomia,' which literally means 'large body'. Babies can grow to 5–5.5 kg (11– 12 lb), which makes diabetic women far more likely to need to have a Caesarean section delivery, or in some cases, for doctors to decide that the baby should be induced early.

There are straightforward ways of measuring a baby while he or she is in the womb, and your doctor will recommend the right method of delivery for you. The reason why it is vital you remain in total control of your blood sugar levels is that, in rare cases, the baby can grow too big too soon and has to be delivered before some vital organs are fully formed.

After the birth, your baby will have to start regulating its own glucose levels, without reference to you. If you have a high blood glucose level prior to labour, your baby could have very low blood sugar immediately after delivery. It is vital that, as a diabetic, you have your baby in hospital rather than at home where your baby's blood sugar levels can be checked within minutes. As the doctors do that, they will also test for low serum calcium and magnesium to make sure everything is normal.

During the birth, your insulin requirements will fall steeply, as the inhibiting hormones will have been removed from your body with the placenta. What is in your system will be able to function efficiently and your need will drop. It might stay low for a few days before returning to pre-pregnancy levels – your doctor will advise you on what action to take.

If you are breastfeeding, you may need to alter your insulin dose as breast milk contains lactose, a type of sugar, so when your baby feeds your blood sugar will drop. Incorporating an extra portion of starchy foods in your healthy eating plan every day can help prevent hypos.

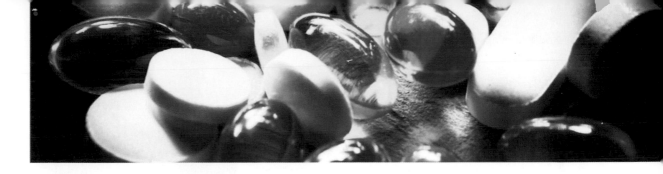

THE DIABETES AND PREGNANCY CHECKLIST

If you're diabetic your pregnancy will be closely monitored and your medicaton adjusted accordingly. With the right care, there's no reason why you can't have a healthy pregnancy.

THERE IS NO REASON AT ALL WHY DIABETIC WOMEN CANNOT CARRY AND DELIVER A PERFECTLY HEALTHY BABY, PROVIDED THEY TAKE EXTRA SPECIAL CARE OF THEMSELVES BEFORE AND DURING THE PREGNANCY.

■ Plan your pregnancy – as a diabetic, you should be in optimum health before you conceive.

■ Lose weight before you conceive. Because you will put on fat as a natural part of your pregnancy, it is important you are not overweight to start with.

■ Consult with your doctor as soon as you think you might be pregnant. Don't wait until you are sure, or until you start attending an antenatal clinic, as you will need advice on how exactly to remain at your healthiest.

■ Test your blood sugar at least six times a day. Test it before and after each meal and last thing at night, with the aim of maintaining controlled levels throughout the pregnancy.

■ See a dietician. At this time, what you eat is vitally important because, while you cannot afford to overindulge in the 'eating for two' tradition, neither can you deny yourself the extra intake you will need.

■ Be prepared for extra visits to the antenatal clinic. As a diabetic you will need extra scans to check on your baby's growth, tighter blood pressure measuring and also monitoring of kidney functions.

■ Make sure your partner fully understands your condition. This requires more than just a casual understanding of diabetes. As you become more tired and less mobile, your partner will need to take a more hands-on involvement in maintaining your – and your baby's – good health (see Dad's Box, page 45).

■ Inform colleagues at work. They will need to be aware of what do if complications occur.

■ Discuss the delivery with your doctor. Because babies born to diabetics are often larger than average, medical opinion varies as to whether they should go full term to a normal vaginal birth, be induced a little early (38 weeks), or instead be delivered by Caesarean section. Get involved in any decisions that may be taken.

■ After the birth, the levels of insulin that you need should return quickly to normal. Do not maintain your specially adjusted intake or you could risk provoking a hypo.

STARFILE

SHARON STONE

"Having either type of diabetes is going to be a struggle for anybody, and it can make my life difficult at times, but it can be beaten inasmuch as you don't have to be a slave to it. Diabetes is as much about controlling your lifestyle as it is about your health. It doesn't take a genius to work out that if you eat properly, exercise and keep regular checks on how your body is functioning, while staying away from the stuff that will do you harm – smoking, drinking and so on – you will be better for it. Sometimes I don't think people are made aware enough of how much they can do for themselves. Every diabetic can do their bit to control their condition."

THE DIABETIC CHILD

UNFORTUNATELY, DIABETES IN CHILDREN IS, ON THE RISE. HOWEVER, IT IS NOT TOO DIFFICULT TO MANAGE AS LONG AS THE YOUNGSTERS CONCERNED UNDERSTAND THEIR CONDITION, AND THEIR PARENTS TAKE A FEW PRECAUTIONS.

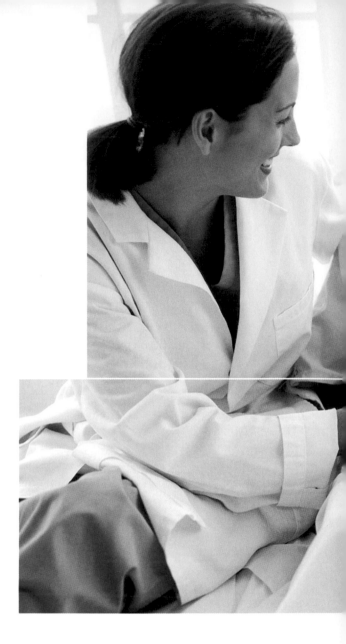

ABOVE ALL ELSE, PARENTS WISH FOR their children to be healthy. So if your son or daughter is diagnosed with diabetes (most likely type I), of course you are going to worry. It can be very distressing to think that one of your children will have to self-inject insulin for the rest of their lives, but kids are amazing, and will probably manage better than you imagine.

Children learn to interpret the world by watching how adults around them react to situations, so if you feel their life will be limited by their diabetes, they will start to think that way too. Remember, there is no way that type I diabetes can be prevented, so you and your child are blameless. Concentrate on teaching your child how best to manage their condition, and don't let it be the thing that dictates your entire family's life. If your child develops diabetes as toddler, they will be too young to understand their condition. They may think the injections are a punishment,

so when it is time for their injections, hold them close and tell them "It's time for your insulin, to make you healthy". Try to turn it into a positive rather than a frightening experience.

Involving children with diabetes in their own care from an early age will help them gain control. If they are too young to self-inject, ask them to chose the spot where you put the needle, or which finger to take a drop of blood from to do a blood sugar test. Discuss what food you are preparing for family meals with them and why, so they learn about the importance of a healthy diet. And let all the family eat the same

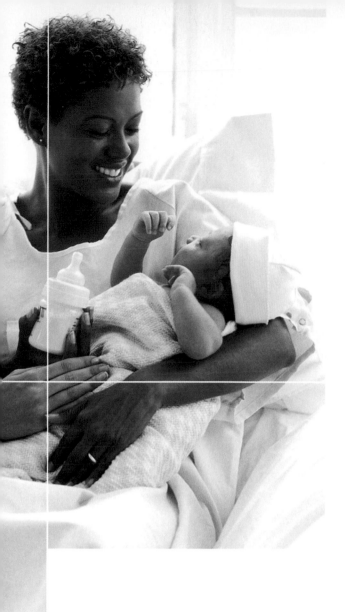

so try not to make their diabetes a source of conflict. Learn to be supportive rather than nagging, and don't try and take over if there are problems. Try to solve them together instead.

If your teenage diabetic wants to go out partying make sure they, and their friends, understand how drinking can affect their diabetes. Alcohol lowers blood sugar, so diabetics should never drink on an empty stomach. A hypo can come on after your teenager has crashed out on a friend's sofa, so he or she should have a snack – even if it's just a packet of crisps, before going to sleep. If your son or daughter has grown up with diabetes they will be acutely aware of how their body reacts to different food and drink, and used to taking responsibility for their own well-being; learning about alcohol should just be one more thing for them to add to their knowledge bank.

Diabetic children at school

One in 700 school children in the UK have diabetes so the chances are someone in your son or daughter's school is also diabetic. Try to find out if this is the case. If your child is diagnosed with diabetes, his or her school should know what to expect. If it doesn't, it's up to you to help his teachers learn about the disease with you.

Children with diabetes need to keep their blood glucose levels constant throughout the day, which means they can't just eat at the school cafeteria at set lunchtimes. Their dietician will suggest eating plans, so take their suggestions along to the school and let the staff know how important it is that your child follows them. If the school rule is 'no eating in the classroom' your child may prefer snacks they can eat between lessons. Their teacher might be happy to let them eat during lessons, but if it makes them feel self-conscious they'll be reluctant to do it. Also, if your child's blood glucose levels are elevated – as can happen if they get a cold – they will probably need to make more trips

things as much as possible so your diabetic child doesn't feel 'different'.

By the time they are old enough to go to secondary school, your child should be able to do their own injections. Depending on their personal care plan, they might need to inject themselves before school and at lunchtime, so make sure they always have all the kit they need with them. Keep talking to them, to make sure they are following their schedule, but make sure they feel responsible for themselves. As they go through adolescence there will be times when parent–child relationships are strained anyhow,

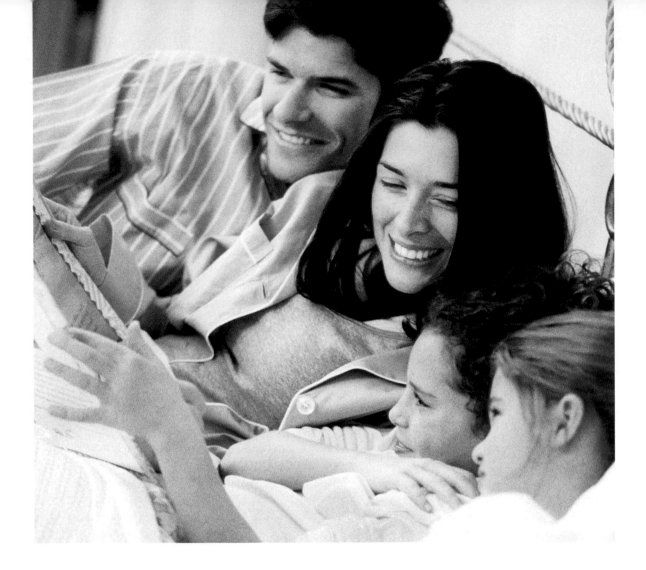

PROTECT YOUR KIDS

Incidences of type II diabetes used to be so rare in people under the age of 35, it was formerly known as adult-onset diabetes. Worryingly, however, this type of diabetes is now on the increase among the young. Fortunately, unlike type I diabetes (which is difficult to head off as its causes have not been nailed down) there is a huge part you can play in reducing your children's risk of contracting type II diabetes.

BE AWARE OF IT AS EARLY AS POSSIBLE

If you have a family history of type II diabetes there are greatly increased chances it will be passed on to your children (see Diabetes Probability panel, p 46). Likewise if you contracted gestational diabetes – even if it didn't remain after the birth. In either case, consult your doctor as soon as possible to talk about having your baby tested.

WATCH YOUR CHILD'S WEIGHT

Just as type II diabetes is linked to being overweight, so the sudden rise of the condition in the young is directly related to the current childhood obesity problem both in the UK and the USA. An overweight child is, as in adulthood, far more likely to contract the disease, so make sure your children follow a healthy eating plan that's suitable for them – growing children have very different dietary requirements to adults – and that they get plenty of exercise.

to the toilet, so make sure their teacher understands that they may have to pop out of the classroom during lessons.

Managed properly, diabetes should not stop a child participating fully in school life, including sports. As long as staff are aware of your child's needs there shouldn't be any problems. Children with diabetes should have an extra snack containing a mix of carbohydrates and protein – a peanut butter sandwich, or a cereal and nut bar – in the morning before their games lesson, or in the afternoon if they are doing after-school sports. No matter what sort of sport they do, they should have a fast-acting sugary snack or drink to hand: they could put a small packet of sweets in their shorts pocket, or a carton of fruit juice by the side of the pool or on the touchline. Leaving them in a bag in the changing rooms means that they are too far away to be of any use if needed.

Make sure the teachers at your child's school know the warning signs of a hypo – drowsiness, sweating, glazed eyes, hunger, irritability, mood swings, shakiness – and what to do if it happens. The first thing to do is get the child to take in some sugar, either a sweet (non-diet) drink or glucose tablets. Whatever happens, keep the channels of communication, between school, child and parent, open, so that you can all play a part in managing your child's diabetes. ◘

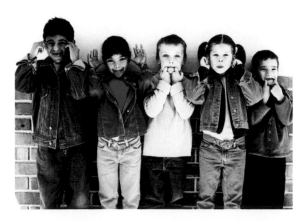

FIND OUT YOUR HISTORY

If you are concerned that your child might be showing symptoms of diabetes, then it's important you find out if there is a history of the condition among either your or your partner's family. Not only will it be seen as a major contributing factor, but it will help your doctor enormously if you can detail any incidences of diabetes among blood relatives.

There is usually no reason why most people shouldn't know their family medical history, and for diabetics it is one more potentially vital aspect to your life. You should ask as many of your blood relatives – parents, siblings, grandparents, aunts, uncles, cousins and so on – as you can if they have had any of the conditions below. Find out when they were diagnosed, what treatment was prescribed and what effect it had on their condition. Compile a record of all of this to discuss with your doctor, as much of it might have a bearing on your or your children's condition and how it is treated. Also find out about other conditions (see below) that may run in your family. Although some of these may appear to have nothing directly to do with diabetes, high blood sugar can result in many different complications including heart disease, nerve problems or circulatory issues. By knowing as much about your genetic history as possible, you doctor will be best informed to detect and deal with anything they come across with you.

DIABETES (TYPES I AND II)
- Heart disease
- High blood pressure
- High cholesterol
- High triglycerides
- Obesity
- Any cancers (what kind, where they originated, where they spread to)
- Alzheimer's disease
- Osteoporosis
- Depression or other psychiatric illnesses

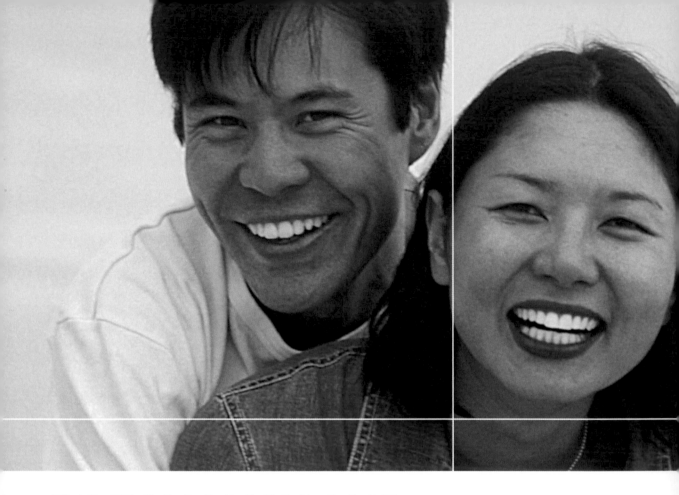

PREGNANCY AND
FAMILY FAQS

IF YOU OR SOMEONE IN YOUR FAMILY HAS BEEN NEWLY DIAGNOSED WITH DIABETES, YOU WILL HAVE PLENTY OF QUESTIONS. NEVER BE TOO EMBARRASSED TO DISCUSS CONCERNS WITH YOUR DOCTOR OR HEALTHCARE TEAM – THEY'RE THERE TO SUPPORT AND HELP YOU.

My daughter has diabetes. Can she still do sports at school?
Of course. Regular exercise is good for everyone's health, including diabetics. She should eat an extra snack before her timetabled games lessons or after-school sports, and always have a sugary snack or drink close at hand during the game in case she has a hypo. Make sure her teachers and coaches know how to recognize the signs of a hypo, and how to treat it.

My son has diabetes, and wants to go away on a Scout camp. Is it OK to let him go?

Yes, providing you are confident he can self-manage his diabetes for the length of the trip without you there. Have a chat with the Scout leader before the camp and make sure there are trained first aiders in the group. Write out a schedule for his injections or tablets so that he can keep

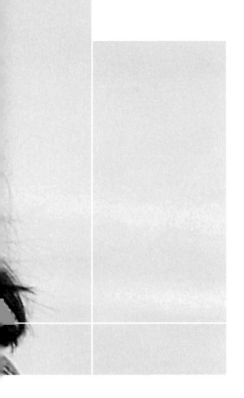

track of his medication. Make sure he has contact details for you and his doctor, so that he can rest assured there will always be someone at the end of the phone if he has concerns.

I've been told by my doctor that I have gestational diabetes. Will it harm my baby?
No, it shouldn't if you get proper treatment and carefully follow the dietary advice you will be given. The most likely problem you face is that any extra blood sugar passing through the placenta will make your baby grow to be very big. While he or she will be no less healthy than if you didn't have gestational diabetes, a normal delivery at 40 weeks could be difficult.

Your doctor will measure your baby in the womb and may recommend that the baby is induced early or that you have a Caesarean section.

Can I breastfeed if I'm diabetic?
Yes, of course, although you may need to adjust the amount of insulin you take. As you will be giving your baby lactose – the sugar found in milk – when you feed him, your own blood sugar will drop. This could prompt a hypo, especially for insulin-dependent mums. Tell your doctor you intend to breastfeed, as he may want to alter your medication accordingly.

My teenage son wants to party all the time, but I'm worried alcohol is bad for his diabetes. Should I tell him not to drink?
No. Forbidding him from drinking will not help him learn how to manage alcohol and his diabetes. The fact that your son wants to go out with his friends and have a drink is normal and shouldn't be a problem, providing he doesn't binge-drink. It's important he knows that alcohol will lower his blood sugar level, and that he has been given advice on how he should cope with that, ie by eating some crisps with his drink. Make sure he has a meal before he goes out, and leave a snack

out for him when he gets home to prevent a hypo later in the night. He should also learn how different drinks will affect him – he should only drink low-calorie mixers and watch out for low-sugar beers and lagers, which tend to be higher in alcohol. Show him that you trust him, and he'll want to live up to that.

My daughter is self-conscious about the marks on her legs from where she injects herself. What should I do?
Unfortunately it's hard to avoid getting bruises at injection sites, and if your daughter is injecting herself several times a day, she's probably going to have quite a few bruises. To minimize bruising, tell her to press firmly with her thumb over the place where she injects immediately after taking out the needle. Two or three minutes' pressure should stop any bleeding under the skin. If she picks sites near the top of her thighs then these shouldn't show when she wears shorts or a short skirt. As it is important to vary injection sites, maybe she could also try using her tummy or buttocks. If she is worried about potential boyfriends, remind her that anyone who genuinely loves her will not be put off by either her diabetes or the bruises.

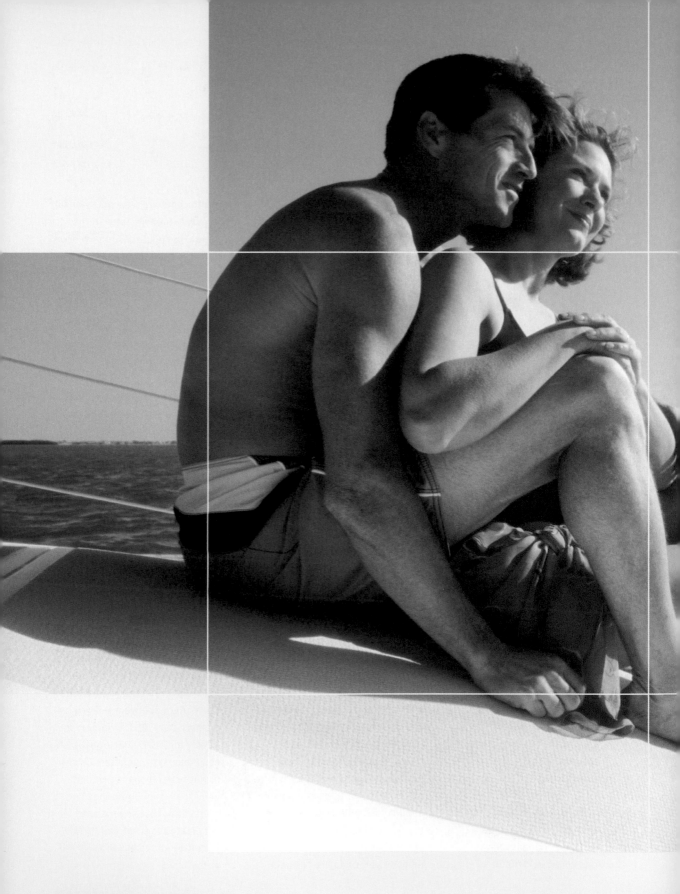

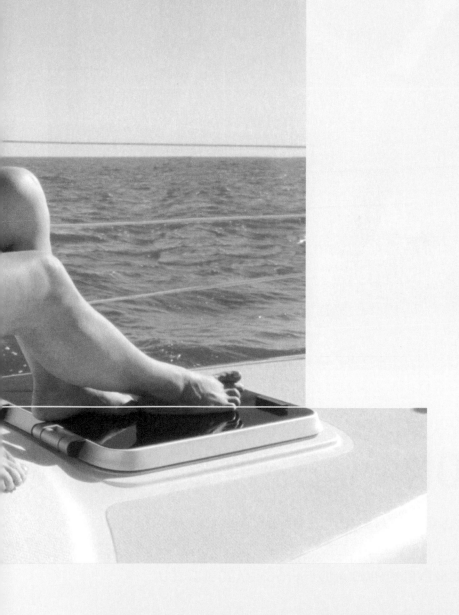

CONTROLLING DIABETES

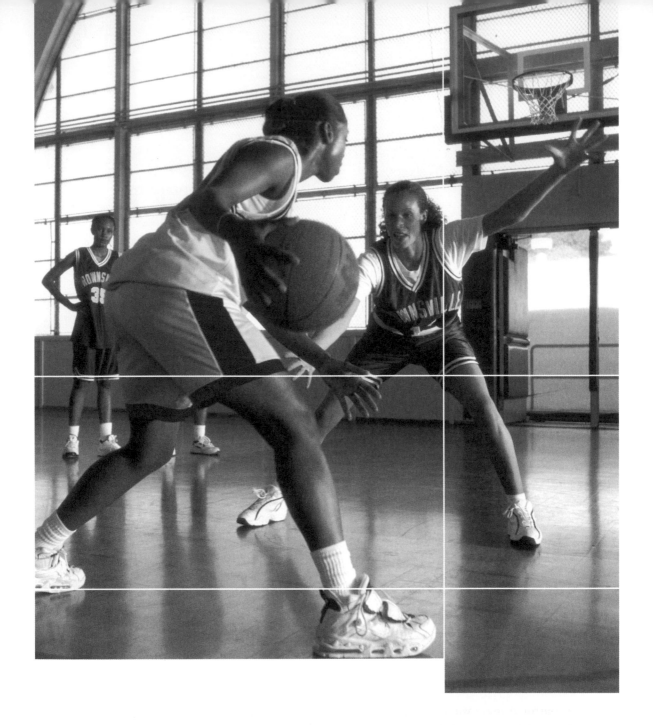

TAKING ON DIABETES

TAKING CONTROL OF YOUR DIABETES AND ITS TREATMENT WILL NOT MEAN CURING IT, BUT IT WILL MAKE YOUR LIFE SO MUCH LESS STRESSFUL AND ENSURE YOU GET THE MAXIMUM BENEFIT FROM EVERYTHING AND EVERYONE AROUND YOU.

NO MATTER HOW SURE YOU THOUGHT you were that you had a form of diabetes, to actually be diagnosed with it is liable to knock you sideways. As your doctor makes you aware of the condition that will change your life and how you live it, it is perfectly natural for you to be focussed on the dangers, the potential problems and the inconveniences of what the future holds. However, once you have fully taken in what you have been told, this moment is also the time in which you can start taking control of this radical new aspect of how you will be living. Just because you aren't going to be able to cure your diabetes, there is no reason why you should ever feel like you are a victim of it.

Taking control of your life from a health and fitness point of view is the whole purpose of the Prevention Health Guides series, and this section will give advice and tips on how to remain in charge of your diabetes.

You will, by now, have been informed of your condition and have reached an understanding of what it is, and so you will be ready to take control. These coming pages will discuss how to do exactly that by using conventional medicine and complementary treatments, through diet and by adopting an exercise routine. Each aspect will allow you to live your life to the fullest while keeping inconvenience and suffering to a minimum; in some cases it will even allow you to overcome certain aspects and symptoms. But before you can outsmart diabetes, you will have to out-think it.

Taking control in your own mind is probably the most important step you will take, post-diagnosis. It signals the start of your fight back, which is a psychological milestone so immense it can actually have physical implications – you will now be much less stressed about your condition and any previous high stress levels could have been making things worse. Be aware that stress switches your body to 'fight or flight' mode, resulting in a surge of blood sugar in anticipation

DE-STRESS FOR DIABETES

You can play a significant part in lowering your blood sugar levels if you de-stress for just 10 minutes a day. First find a quiet spot where you are likely to be undisturbed (you will never de-stress if you feel self-conscious or are worrying about being interrupted): this might be going for a walk, sitting in your car or simply shutting your office door. Close your eyes and focus on breathing deeply and slowly. Acknowledge any thoughts that might pop into your head, but don't dwell on them and get back to concentrating on your breathing. Keep this up for between five and ten minutes, and take time out to do it a couple of times a day.

of some form of action. Once you are feeling more relaxed, you can begin to look at your situation logically and make sure you have the upper hand.

Firstly you shouldn't feel at all embarrassed about your diabetes. Talk to your family, friends and colleagues about it, as you will need their support and maybe, in certain situations, their help. When you go to visit your doctor, take somebody with you if you want to. As well as the moral support, this will give you something of a strength-in-numbers advantage, and a companion could prove useful when it comes to understanding what was said by your doctor once you have left the building. Should your doctor object to you bringing somebody with you, then you might consider getting a new doctor. See the feature on page 73 for advice on the conversation you should be having with your doctor.

Next there are certain logistic aspects with which you will need to get to grips. If you have to take insulin you need to work out a routine, and practise with the needle – this might involve conquering a major fear, but at least that can be ▶

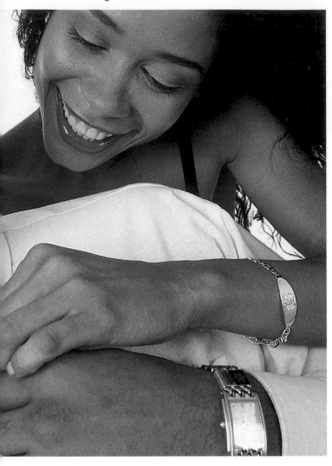

A medical identity bracelet informs people that you are diabetic and ensures you are given the right care in an emergency – there is a wide range of jewellery available

held up as a huge achievement on your part. With the different types of insulin there are on the market (see page 71), you might actually have some choice in the matter, so it is well worth a conversation with your doctor. Likewise, taking glucose-lowering pills if you have to, work to build a routine that causes as little inconvenience as possible. In both cases, it can help enormously if you involve your children in this, there is nothing kids love more than to have to remind adults they should be doing something. But don't actually count on them to be consistently reliable monitors as they do have a great deal of other things to think about!

Now you are making the decisions yourself, or even if you are not you are contributing to them. Such an approach at such an early stage will allow you to continue in a proactive frame of mind. Of course it is going to be tough to see any actual advantages of being a diabetic, but there are certainly a few positives you can accentuate as you continue to take control. Like the major lifestyle changes you should be making, especially if you are a type II diabetic and you need to keep your blood sugar levels down.

Although you might be being told to change to a healthy eating plan and take up a form of exercise, don't see it as some sort of punishment. Look on it as a bonus. For a start healthy eating doesn't mean boring eating, as our selection of mouth-watering recipes (see pp 124-155) proves, and to make this change is something that would be of benefit to anybody, diabetic or otherwise. Taking regular exercise brings its own rewards too, inasmuch as the increase in cardiovascular levels will make you feel so much better. These adjustments to your lifestyle will make you feel better, live more actively, lose weight and look much better. Now how good is that? ◘

DIABETIC BLING

It is essential for diabetics to carry identification because in an emergency, they will need those around them to become aware of their condition as quickly as possible. Traditionally, the most effective way of doing this is with a diabetic's bracelet or medallion, and, equally traditionally, this jewellery has all the élan you'd expect from what it is – a medical identity tag. But it doesn't have to be like that. There are many specialist jewellery firms that produce wide ranges of stylish diabetic identification products, and there is nothing stopping you choosing your own and getting it engraved with your detail at your local jeweller's, or get some custom-made identity bling for those special occasions. After all, it's you has to wear it so you ought to be as in control of that as you are with the rest of your jewellery box.

TAKING CONTROL OF DIABETES

1) GET CONFIRMATION OF WHETHER YOU HAVE IT OR NOT

Go and see your doctor or a health-care professional, and ask to be tested for diabetes. If the tests are positive, make sure you get your blood sugar, blood pressure and cholesterol checked. You should also get a foot and eye examination. Take a friend with you to your appointment if you want to.

2) TAKE TIME TO FULLY DIGEST WHAT YOU HAVE BEEN TOLD

If you are diagnosed as diabetic, make sure you fully absorb what you have been told. Don't make assumptions or hasty decisions. The only way you will take control of your situation is with a clear head.

3) FIND OUT THE FACTS FOR YOURSELF

Make sure you are in possession of all the information available to you. Look on the Internet, go to your local library or contact one of the many organizations (see page 156). In this case it's true that knowledge really is power.

4) WORK OUT HOW THOSE FACTS APPLY TO YOU

Once you've gained a good all round understanding of diabetes, focus on the particular type that you have, and with this knowledge work out how you can make your life easier. You could be surprised at how much difference being fully prepared can make.

5) PREPARE YOURSELF FOR YOUR NEXT CONVERSATION WITH YOUR DOCTOR

When you go to see your doctor, you should aim to be in the position of being able to answer practically any question you might ask! Arrive armed with information and you will know if you are being sold short or misdiagnosed. There is no reason why your doctor shouldn't welcome your contributions. Also, if you know what you want to talk about you will probably get a much better service.

6) ACCENTUATE THE POSITIVES

It might not, at first, seem that there are too many. But if being diabetic means you can no longer carry on making excuses for not eating healthily or doing exercise, then that has to be a bonus.

7) START MAKING LIFESTYLE CHANGES

Don't let diabetes change you. Go forward with whatever adjustments you have to make to your life with gusto and as if they were your idea. Think they are only being made to improve your quality of life.

8) DON'T WORRY

Stress can only make your condition worse, as it can trigger surges in blood sugar. And besides, worrying never changed anything!

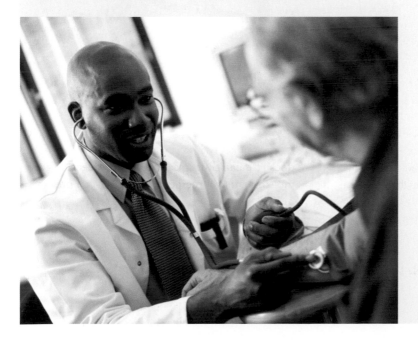

DIABETES DEVELOPMENTS

THE FIGHT TO CONTROL DIABETES NEVER STOPS, AND ALL OVER THE WORLD SCIENTISTS AND RESEARCHERS ARE RACING TO BRING YOU THE LATEST DEVELOPMENTS. WE'VE ROUNDED UP THE BEST OF THEM AND THROWN IN SOME HANDY TIPS.

SUPER CINNAMON

Scientists in America have made a great discovery – by accident! While researching how different sorts of foods affected blood sugar levels, they were astonished to find that the American classic, apple pie, actually helped. The reason: cinnamon.

Further investigations from the US Agricultural Research Service and colleagues in research institutes in Peshawar, Pakistan, have confirmed that having half a teaspoon of cinnamon a day significantly reduces blood sugar levels in people with diabetes, and in those who have a blood sugar problem but are unaware of it. Cinnamon contains MCHP, a water-soluble polyphenol compound that mimics insulin. It not only lowers blood sugar levels, but can help lower levels of fats and 'bad' cholesterol – both of which are controlled, in part, by insulin. Volunteers with type II diabetes were given cinnamon capsules to take after meals, and the effects were noticeable within weeks, with an average 20 per cent drop in blood sugar. But when the volunteers stopped taking the capsules, their levels began to creep up again. This is great news,

but be warned – it's not an excuse to eat Chelsea buns or apple pie. The trick is to add cinnamon to a normal, healthy diet. Try having stewed or baked fruit, or even a cinnamon stick in your tea.

THE TRUTH IS IN THE THIGHS

How a child grows in the womb and in the first years of life can indicate how healthy it will be throughout its life. Now scientists have drawn a link between thigh length – a good indicator of healthy childhood growth – and the chances of developing diabetes in later life for

certain parts of the population, especially Caucasian women. For every 1 cm (0.4 in) less than average thigh length, the women studied were 19 per cent more likely to be diabetic, and also at a higher risk of glucose intolerance, the precursor to diabetes. Some 8,700

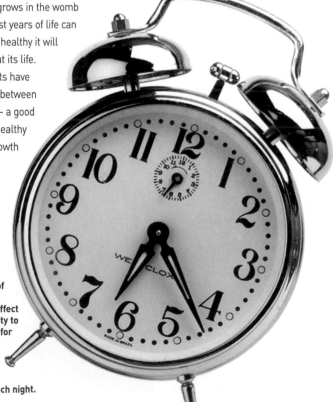

The amount of sleep you get can directly affect your sensitivity to insulin – aim for eight hours and try to go to bed at around the same time each night.

people of both sexes and varied ethnic origins took part in the study. The scientific team found that the average thigh length for people with normal glucose tolerance was 40.2 cm (15.8 in), but only 38.3 cm (15 in) among women with diabetes.

The scientists believe that poor nutrition, both for the foetus in the womb and during early infancy, can have a huge impact on health in later life. Other studies have also linked low birth weight with heart disease and diabetes.

SLEEP IT OFF

Researchers have already proved conclusively that by not getting enough sleep you are damaging your insulin sensitivity. Numerous studies have shown that people who got less than six hours sleep were 40 per cent less sensitive than those who got their full eight hours.

However, studies have now shown that regular sleeping patterns – going to bed and getting up at the same time every day – can also help combat insulin insensitivity, as the body settles into natural rhythms of hormonal production.

CALM DOWN, CALM DOWN

We've all told our children that getting angry and frustrated isn't good for their health, and now here's the proof. Hostile behaviour has been linked to 'metabolic syndrome', a collection of risk factors including obesity, high blood pressure and insulin resistance, which all point towards diabetes and heart disease. Certain personality types have long been suspected to be more vulnerable to heart disease, and this study of children and teenagers – conducted over a three-year period – fits the theory. The children that were hostile – easily angered, cynical and untrusting – were three times more likely to develop metabolic syndrome than their more tranquil classmates.

STEM CELL SCIENCE

Cutting edge stem cell research carried out at King's College, London, has offered new hope of a cure for type I diabetes in the future. Scientists have discovered that it is possible to 'switch on' the genes in stem cells (the cells that come from human embryos) that produce hormones in the pancreas, including the genes that are involved in insulin production. It's still a long way from being a cure, but it certainly shows that a cure might be possible in the future.

We all know that maintaining a healthy weight is a vital step in the treatment and control of type II diabetes, but a new study has shown it is potentially life-saving. Data from 44,000 diabetics was analysed in the research, which concluded that being overweight could reduce the life expectancy of a type II sufferer by eight years, and that having a high body mass index (BMI) is a leading cause of premature death in people who have diabetes. ▶

WRITE IT DOWN

One of the best ways to get started on the weight loss trail is also one of the simplest – write down everything you eat, where you eat it and with whom.

Don't include just meals, but also every snack or nibble or drink (other than water) that passes your lips. Keep this food diary for a whole week, then sit down and assess what you have consumed during the previous seven days as an overview. Your consumption will appear very different when you look at it like that, as so much of the stuff you don't usually notice you're eating – the incidental 'grazing' you do when you're offered a biscuit or that after-dinner mint – will have been written down and will now be given in evidence against you! You might actually find it quite shocking and it should go a long way to pushing you into changing what you eat.

A detailed food diary will also help you take control of eating habits you might not even be aware you have. Keeping a record of the times and the places you eat allows you to identify patterns and change them if you find you frequently eat badly in certain situations. Writing down who you eat it with means you will be aware of just who are the bad influences on you, and that you can prepare yourself to eat the right things when you go out for a meal with them.

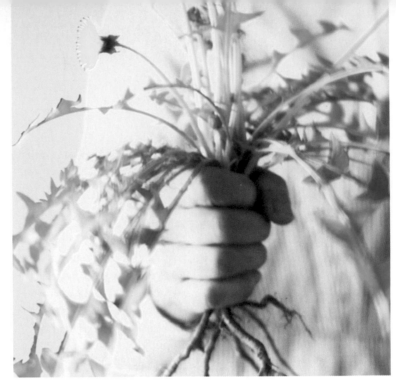

Dandelion stimulates the liver to store and release glucose more efficiently – it can be eaten as salad leaves, and the roots can be drunk as a tea.

DANDELION DISCOVERY

Dandelion roots can help normalize blood sugar levels and reduce the free radical damage that can contribute to diabetes-related problems such as heart disease and eye disorders. The way to make use of the roots is as tea, brewing a pot of three teaspoons of dried dandelion root in a pint of boiling water. Let it steep for 10 minutes before straining.

CUT BACK ON COFFEE

In one study involving a dozen people without diabetes, researchers found that the amount of caffeine in two cups of strong coffee reduced insulin sensitivity by 15 per cent. Decreased insulin sensitivity is a risk factor for type II diabetes, and the researchers think this may have serious implications for diabetics. If you drink a lot of coffee and have difficulty controlling your diabetes, it may be worth cutting down your caffeine intake and talking to your doctor about it.

FIND OUT IF YOU SNORE

If you snore every night, you really should get tested for diabetes. Recent studies in the USA seem to show a link between snoring and risk of diabetes. A study of 7,000 nurses found that those who snored every night had more than twice the normal risk of developing type II diabetes. This wasn't anything to do with obesity, as the chances of becoming diabetic were the same regardless of how much each subject weighed. Snoring triggers an increase in hormones called catecholamines, which seem to be linked to insulin resistance, a precursor to diabetes. Sleep apnoea, a condition in which you actually stop breathing during the night, may also have the same effect.

So if you snore every night and you're also overweight, see your doctor. A simple blood test will determine if you are diabetic or not, and it may help your quality of life in general to discuss ways to control the snoring.

ANTIOXIDANTS

'Antioxidant' is a medical buzzword at the moment, not just in diabetes treatment but in complementary medicine

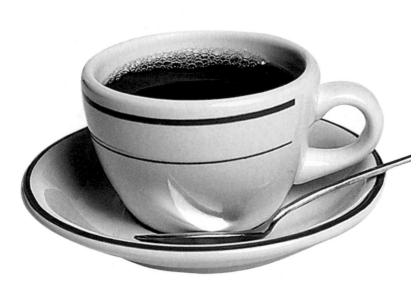

Caffeine has been found to decrease sensitivity to insulin, so if you're diabetic opt for decaffeinated alternatives to regular coffee and tea

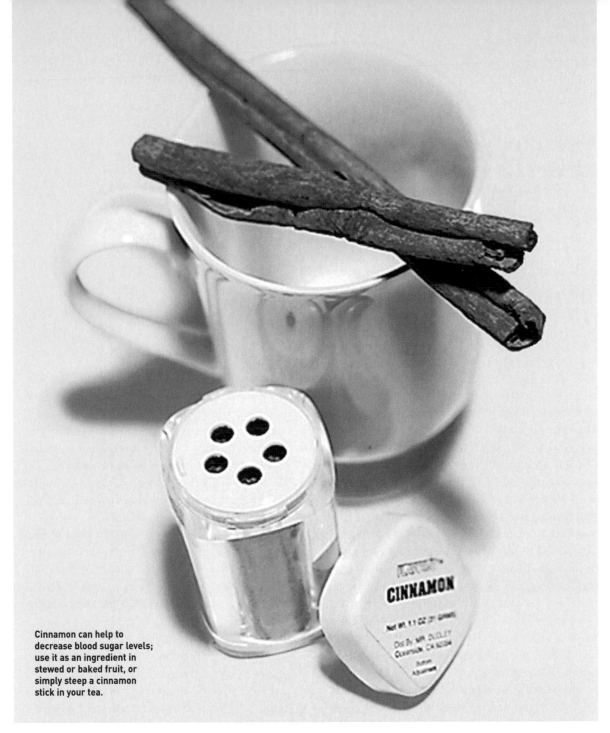

Cinnamon can help to
decrease blood sugar levels;
use it as an ingredient in
stewed or baked fruit, or
simply steep a cinnamon
stick in your tea.

in general, yet few people really know what it means. In simple terms, antioxidants are plant chemical substances used by the body to protect itself against free radicals. They also help to neutralize free radical damage experienced by people with abnormal metabolism due to their diabetes.

We've already mentioned the polyphenols that occur in cinnamon, but there are others. For example, green tea extract contains powerful antioxidants such as catechin.

Recent research suggests that catechins can improve glucose and lipid metabolism, and may be helpful for people with Insulin Resistance Syndrome, which is linked with the development of type II diabetes. You can get the benefits from drinking green tea steeped in hot, but not boiling water (which will make the tea bitter and destroy some of the antioxidants). ◨

DIABETES AND THE OVERWEIGHT

WHILE OBESITY IS SEEN AS A MAJOR FACTOR IN TYPE II DIABETES, WEIGHT
LOSS SHOULD BE AN AIM FOR EVERY DIABETIC WHO IS OVERWEIGHT.

AS THE VAST MAJORITY OF DIABETICS are type II, and a large proportion of those are overweight. Although all fat people are not diabetic and not all diabetics are fat, tests have proved that, in a significant number of cases, the increased weight someone may be carrying is directly related to an increase in blood sugar levels. The fasting norm for somebody of the right weight for their height ought to be 115 mg/dl (115 milligrams of sugar in every decilitre of blood), but for the obese individual the fasting norm is more likely to be measured at up to 150 mg/dl, enough to be considered diabetic. The same test has also shown that to lose weight will bring these blood sugar levels down accordingly.

Quite apart from just taking more sugar on board through overeating, another cause of these higher than normal levels is that overweight people actually need to produce proportionately more insulin to manage their blood glucose, and even then it does not function as efficiently. This is due to extra body fat increasing a condition known as insulin resistance, which, remarkably, would appear to have its cause in the body itself trying to stop a person overeating. As increases in blood sugar due to overeating cause a demand for extra insulin to cope with it, so the raised blood insulin levels set off an internal alarm and actually cause a reduction in the insulin receptors in the

cell walls (the areas insulin attaches to, allowing sugar to be absorbed). Consequently, the pancreas goes into overdrive, but the more insulin it produces, the more efficient the insulin resistance becomes. And the levels of blood glucose, already high, become dangerously so. It is not fully understood why this occurs in fat people, but it is commonly thought to be a warning shot, telling whoever it is to stop eating so much.

Of course it's not simply a matter of how much overweight people eat that affects their blood sugar, but what they eat and when they eat it. Essentially, the body eats for nutrients and will stop feeling hungry once sufficient nutrients have been taken on board, but in today's world too much food is devoid of these necessary nutrients. Thus while so much food has some calorific value – fuel – it isn't serving the body's greater needs and hunger strikes long before the empty calories have been burnt off. More nutritionally devoid food is taken on for the calories alone and the obesity icicle is in place.

When you eat is also crucial. It is not good for a diabetic to eat one or two huge meals a day, as it encourages blood sugar peaks and troughs. Again there is a link here to being overweight as so many obese people eat a lot once or twice a day instead of the recommended little and often. Five small meals a day or frequent snacks ▶

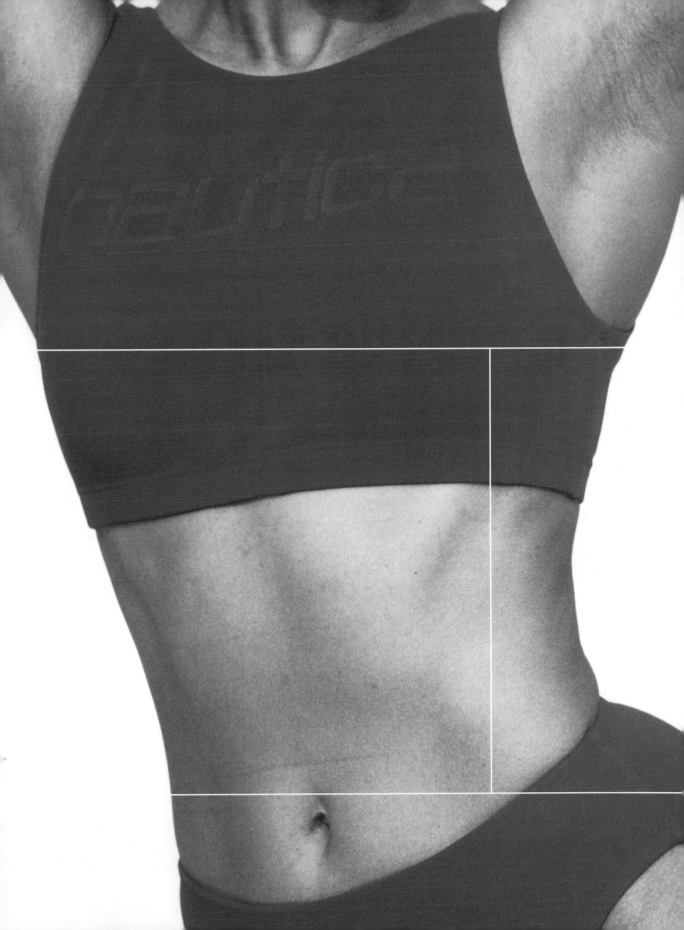

of fruit or wholemeal goods are ideal. Amazingly, losing as little as 4.5 kg (10 lbs) could significantly improve your insulin function and lower your blood sugar levels, which will go a long way to putting you in control of your type II diabetes. Then if you only suffer from mild diabetes, sometimes known as Impaired Glucose Tolerance, reducing your body weight by as little as 5 per cent can lower your risk of getting regular diabetes by as much as a massive 80 per cent.

Weight loss isn't really that hard to get control of either. Once you have arrived at the combination of diet and exercise that best suits you, set targets for yourself that are at once attainable and significant. Losing 1.4 kg (3 lb) a week, for instance, is relatively easy and may not seem like much, but keep it up every week for a month and you will have lost nearly 6.4 kg (1 stone). Carry on for another month and you'll double the loss. And you will notice the results immediately by getting through the day with renewed energy, and every time you glance in a mirror. Not only are you beating diabetes but you are making yourself look and feel better at the same time. ◻

THE LOW CARB SOLUTION

Carb lowering is one of the best ways for a diabetic to lose weight. Largely because if you eat too many grams of quickly absorbed carbohydrates (foods with a high glycaemic index, see page 112) you will flood your bloodstream with sugar. Since your blood will then contain more sugar than you will need for energy it will be stored as fat. When this happens, your blood sugar level drops, leaving you hungry again. Fluctuating blood sugar levels make it difficult for insulin to do its job. Ideally, you should be consuming 45–75 g (1.6–2.6 oz) of carbohydrate per meal and 15–30 g (0.5–1 oz) per snack, and you should have three of each every day.

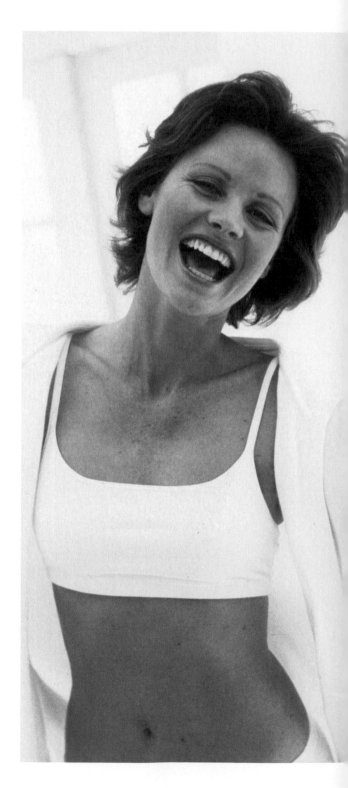

THE EASY WAY TO LOSE THAT WEIGHT

Whatever exercise and eating plan you opt for as you take control of your diabetes by losing weight, you always benefit from some extra help. These basic principles can be applied to any option you choose and will certainly make your weight loss life a whole lot easier.

ALWAYS EAT WHEN YOU'RE HUNGRY

Really, people should eat every two to four hours, which means having four or five smaller meals a day. To follow the modern tendency to eat only one or two meals a day means that during the day you will override the part of your brain that tells you when you are hungry and also when you are full. As a result, you end up overeating when you do finally sit down. You wouldn't run your car until it is past empty, then fill it up so that it overflows, would you? Then why do the same thing to your body? Missing meals or starving yourself in the name of weight loss will always backfire on you and could end up making you gain weight. If it isn't convenient to have extra meals during the course of your day, you should make sure you have a constant supply of healthy snack foods available to you.

STOP EATING WHEN YOU ARE FULL

It may seem obvious, but the recent trend for bigger portions means so many of us have for a long time been overriding the signals that tell us when we are full . So long, in fact that we have forgotten what they are, hence we need to make the effort to start focussing on them again. One of the ways to pay attention to these signs is to eat much slower. Such is the pace of life that we tend to eat a great deal faster than people did a decade or so ago and as it takes about 20 minutes for our brains to register how much we are eating. It is so easy to eat past the point of being full quite literally without realizing. Don't loosen your belt halfway through a big dinner – if it is too tight, it is because you've eaten enough.

HAVE A GOOD BREAKFAST

This really is the most important meal of the day as it helps you avoid overeating later on – people who don't eat breakfast are far more likely to be overweight than those who do. Opt for breakfast foods that will give you protein and a little fat in addition to carbs and sugar. They will give you the slow-release energy you need to get through the morning. But don't fill up on sugary breakfast cereal, as it will only last you for about half an hour and then you will be hungry all over again.

COUNT CALORIES NOT JUST FAT

Although fat has more calories than protein or carbohydrate foods, - nine per gram for fat vs four per gram for carbs – low fat foods can often be deceptive. Sure they may be, as their labels say, low in fat, but the chances are they will be so loaded with carbohydrate they will actually contain more calories than you need. And definitely more than you should be getting if you're trying to lose weight!

FILL UP ON FIBRE

Fibre-rich foods are a weight loss dream. They are filling, metabolism-boosting and come complete with lots of vitamins, minerals and nutrients. And they are more or less devoid of fat.

CHECK YOUR PORTION SIZES

While it goes without saying that if you are trying to lose weight you shouldn't be super-sizing anything, you will also need to pay attention to what else you are eating. We are eating and expecting increasingly bigger portions – in restaurants, in fast food outlets, in packaged food. Don't feel obliged to finish everything that is put in front of you. And avoid buying the larger packets that are on the shelves these days – you'll be less tempted to overeat if you opt for the smaller options.

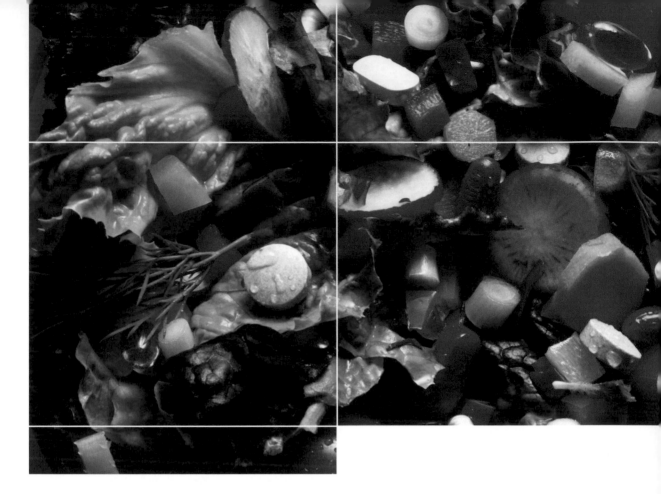

CONTROLLING DIABETES
THROUGH MEDICATION

PRESCRIPTIVE MEDICINE PLAYS A HUGE PART IN CONTROLLING DIABETES,
AND IT IS VITAL YOU UNDERSTAND WHAT YOU ARE TAKING.

ALTHOUGH A HEALTHY EATING AND physical fitness plan is vital for you as a diabetic, it's likely that your doctor will put you on some sort of medication. If you are a type I diabetic you will immediately be put on a course of insulin, as your body produces none of its own. As this means you will be unable to convert the glucose in your body into fuel, you will have to take insulin from an outside source and that will mean daily injections for the rest of your life. There is, at the moment, no alternative.

If your diabetes is type II, you may not be put on medication, as it may be possible to manage your blood sugar with a combination of careful monitoring, healthy diet and regular exercise. But either because your insulin production is low or because your body is unable to use it efficiently, the result may be either the overproduction of blood glucose or some glucose staying unused in your system. Either way, your doctor may feel this is too serious to be controlled with lifestyle changes, so will prescribe tablets.

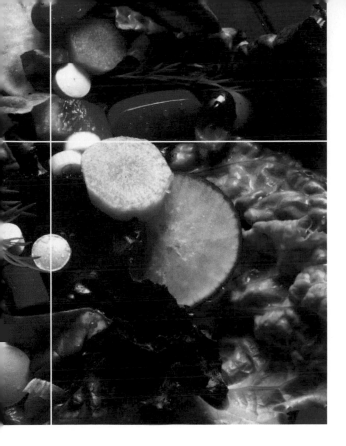

If you need to use either form of medication to assist in controlling your diabetes, it is important to know exactly what it is you are taking, and precisely why it has been prescribed. The box on page 73 gives guidelines of how you should approach a meeting with your doctor and what questions you should ask. Before you even get to the surgery, though, it will help you enormously if you make sure you know in advance what kinds of medication you may be offered.

Insulin

Insulin was discovered in the 1920s and it revolutionized the treatment and care of diabetics. For years, the insulin injected was produced by cattle or pigs, but recently it has become one of genetic engineering's success stories and enough 'human' insulin is now produced in laboratories to meet worldwide demands.

There are two types of insulin in use: slow-acting and fast-acting. The former has its actions slowed down by the addition of different elements or by being treated in a certain way, and a single injection can last up to 24 hours. ▶

LIFE WITHOUT NEEDLES

Injecting insulin is a part of many diabetics' daily routine. And while it's vital to their continued good health, it can still prove inconvenient if not downright painful. As a result, scientific research is being devoted to developing a viable alternative to the potential discomfort of injections a day or of having to wear an insulin pump. The following needle-free alternatives are currently being tested:

ORAL INSULIN SPRAYS
This experimental spray works by spraying an insulin solution into the mouth where it is taken into the bloodstream through the absorbent membranes. In tests, it has proved to work as efficiently as injected insulin in both type I and type II diabetics, particularly in those type II diabetics who did not react to the medication that makes the body's cells more sensitive to insulin.

INSULIN INHALERS
Like an asthmatic's inhaler, these deliver a blast of dry insulin into the lungs, where it is absorbed. In tests in the USA, among type II diabetics, this method proved more effective than injecting. However, over time, the people tested proved far more likely to develop antibodies to insulin, so reducing the hormone's effectiveness.

INSULIN PILLS
For a long time, scientists have been unable to get past the problem of stomach enzymes breaking the insulin down before it can have any effect. However, current research has found a way to surround each insulin molecule with a protective compound to allow it time to do its job. Tests are proving insulin pills to be particularly efficient in controlling blood sugar after meals.

INSULIN SKIN PATCHES
These are still in very early stages of research, but scientists are working to apply nicotine patch technology to the delivery of a controlled dose of insulin.

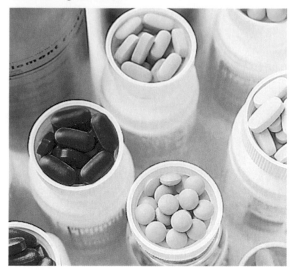

Stay in control of your healthcare by finding out what medication you are being given and why – it's important to understand how what you're taking will improve your condition.

Slow-acting insulins work differently in different people – some need just one shot per day, others may need two, but your doctor will make himself responsible for putting you on the most suitable variety of insulin.

Fast-acting insulin takes effect within only 30 minutes and remains effective, in most people, for around four hours. This is why users need several shots a day. It's not unusual for diabetics to incorporate fast-acting insulin into their diabetes control by injecting just before meals in order to deal with their body's increased demand for insulin when they have eaten.

Glucose-lowering pills

You will only be prescribed glucose-lowering pills if you have type II diabetes. This form of medication has been available for around 50 years and is necessary for the more serious cases of type II diabetes.

When the pancreas either doesn't produce enough insulin for the body's needs or the body cannot make use of it as fuel, the liver gets signals that it is not putting out enough and goes into overdrive, trying to keep up with the apparent demand. This leads to escalating levels of blood glucose, which are sometimes too much to be managed with diet.

There are several different types of glucose-lowering pills on the market and there are as many different ways in which they work to control your levels. Sulphonylureas keeps your blood sugar down by boosting insulin production so it can help blood glucose feed into the body's cells. Biguanides increase glucose's own efficiency levels meaning it is much less reliant on insulin to do its job. Thiazolidinediones make what insulin you do produce work far more effectively, to keep the blood sugar moving through your system. And then there are the many varieties of tablets taken at mealtimes, to deal with the spike in blood sugar that comes after eating.

If you are to be prescribed glucose-lowering pills, your doctor will assess your needs in relation to your insulin production and efficiency capabilities, but be sure you know what it is you are being given and why.

The biggest risk with glucose-lowering medication is the obvious one – it could lower your levels too far and bring on a hypo. Symptoms are dizziness, sweating, an accelerated heartbeat and confused thinking, and you will have to take glucose on board immediately. This is why, when you are prescribed glucose-lowering pills, your doctor should instruct you to always carry glucose tablets or a sugary drink – it may not have made sense at the time, but he or she should have explained that it is an important preventitive precaution. ◘

ASK YOUR DOCTOR ABOUT YOUR MEDICATION

If your doctor opts to manage your diabetes by prescribing medication, make sure you know exactly what it is you are being asked to take, why and what it actually does. This is an important psychological aspect, as deciding your prescription is not a step you can take or, in most cases, even be consulted on. Only by fully understanding what you are being given can you feel like you are retaining control of your treatment. Once you have been given a pre-scription, go through the following checklist with your doctor:

WHAT ARE YOU BEING GIVEN?
Find out the name of the drug being prescribed and the trade names of what you are likely to be given. Ask for this to be written down for you.

WHAT DO THEY ACTUALLY DO?
Don't be palmed off with something as bland as "They'll lower your blood sugar" or "They'll help you produce insulin". Find out scientifically how the drugs you are being prescribed actually work to influence your condition.

WHAT, IF ANY, ARE THE PROBABLE AND POSSIBLE SIDE EFFECTS?
It is just as important to know what might happen as well as what will happen.

WHAT HAPPENS IF YOU TAKE TOO MUCH OR TOO LITTLE OF YOUR MEDICATION?
Although you will be informed of your daily dosage, make sure you fully understand the consequences of accidentally taking too much or too little. This is more than what the symptoms are, but information you need to stay in control.

WHAT ARE THE EARLIEST WARNING SIGNS?
These are vital, as if you have forgotten to take your dosage or have accidentally taken it twice you will be unaware and therefore need to recognize the possibility as early as possible.

WHAT SHOULD YOU AND THOSE AROUND YOU DO?
Clearly understood emergency procedures could be crucial, so get your doctor to run through these in the clearest of terms.

WHEN SHOULD I TAKE MY MEDICATION AND WHY?
It is vital you understand the theory of why you need to take certain medication at certain times. Your life will always be unpredictable, so you will need to understand exactly how the medication works in different circumstances – for example, on an empty stomach or a full stomach or before or after sleep or activity. With this knowledge, you will be better able to improvize if necessary.

DON'T BE SHY TO ASK FOR A SECOND OPINION.
Once you have all the detailed answers from your doctor as to why you are being put on certain medication – and there's no reason at all why you shouldn't be told – get them checked out, against your condition, by somebody else, if for no other reason than to put your mind completely at rest.

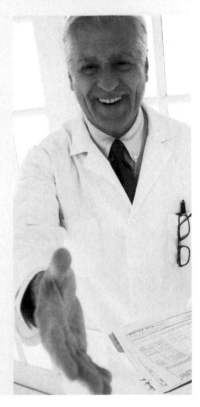

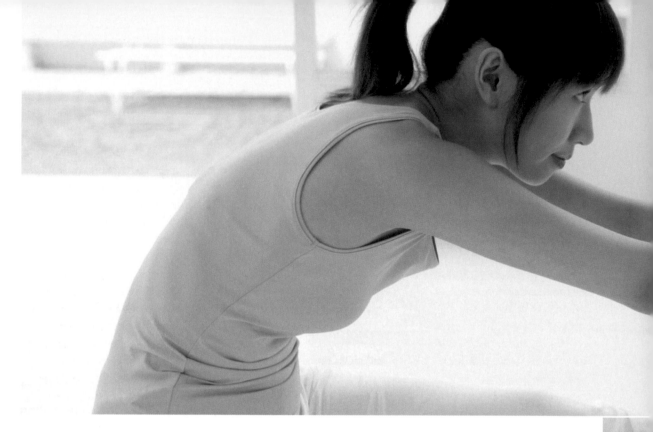

THE COMPLEMENTARY APPROACH

THE BALANCED OPTION OF A HEALTHY DIET, A NUTRITIONAL SUPPLEMENT PLAN, REGULAR EXERCISE AND QUALITY RELAXATION CAN HELP MANAGE TYPE I DIABETES AND MAY EVEN AVOID THE ONSET OF TYPE II.

PREVENTION IS BETTER THAN CURE, it is said, and nowhere more so than with your health. If you think you stand a high chance of developing diabetes, now is the time to act using everything you can.

Professor Jayne Goddard, a qualified homeopath and hypnotherapist and President of the Complementary Medical Association (CMA) says "Because diabetics are at such high risk of complications, and complementary medicine is aimed at preventing, rather than just treating,

I recommend using them to address current symptoms, and also to ward off further complications and conditions like kidney problems, heart disease, vision loss, stroke and nerve damage."

Nutritional therapist and lecturer Antony Haynes agrees. He says as many as one in six of the major causes of insulin resistance is a lack of vital nutrients, including vitamins and minerals. "I see it in my practice all the time. It's the price often paid by a stress-ridden modern lifestyle. Once, of course, we were seasoned hunter-

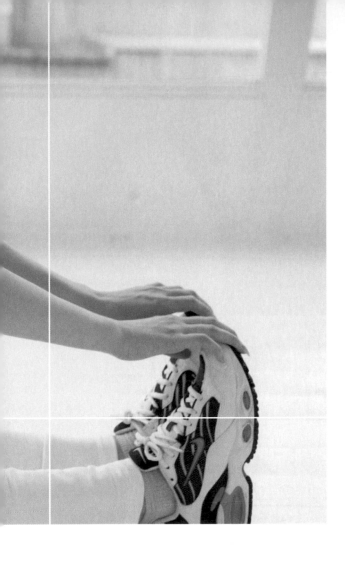

micronutrients, many of which are now depleted within our diet, and problems particularly arise with mineral deprivation. According to a study by mineralogist and nutritionist David Thomas, micronutrient levels in the soil are so severely depleted it is having a drastic effect on what is being grown. His findings include alarming results for both chromium and magnesium (levels down by 75 per cent in the past 60 years). Chromium is highly regarded in its role in helping to balance blood sugar levels according to Antony Haynes. "A diet high in refined carbohydrates, grains and sugars will deplete your chromium intake by as much as 97 per cent. Not only that, a person with this kind of diet increases the excretion of chromium from the body by as much as 300 per cent," he states. What better reason do we need for mineral supplementation to complement the diet?

Sadly many people develop life-threatening conditions because their diabetes is diagnosed too late. Diagnosing diabetes early means that it can be treated and the risk of developing serious complications can be greatly reduced. In an ideal world the best form of therapy for diabetes is prevention itself. But think positive; it's never too late to start a holistic wellbeing regime of optimum nutrition, exercise and relaxation.

Before you embark on a mind, body and soul campaign, check out the Complementary Medical Association website (see page 156) to find a qualified practitioner. Be aware though that just because a remedy works on a friend or colleague, it won't necessarily benefit you. No two people or symptoms are alike, so consult a therapist who will look at you and your case individually.

Also, and this is crucial, check with your doctor and nutritionist or therapist to identify any contra-indications with existing medication (prescription or otherwise) or medical conditions before you embark on either a supplement or mind-body course. ▶

gatherers, primed to flight or fight for survival, but times have changed. Now we have status and achievement anxiety, a sedentary work style and prepared food full of fat, sugar and salt. This is why, in the shrinking world of the past 60 years or so, migrant races have become so vulnerable to diabetes – they've abandoned the indigenous diet of their forefathers."

Indeed, figures from Diabetes UK reveal that people of African-Caribbean or South Asian origin are three to five times more likely to develop diabetes than white members of the population.

If you look closer at how we live today and what happens – or doesn't happen – to the food we eat before it arrives at our tables, it isn't really all that surprising that experts like Professor Goddard and Antony Haynes are so concerned. Glucose control depends on a wide range of

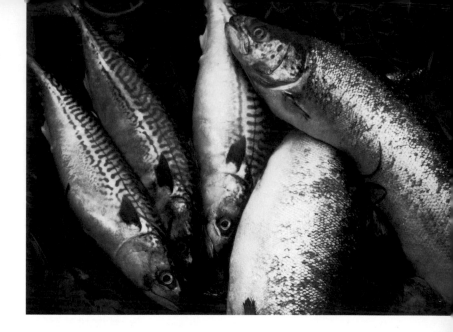

GLUCOSE TOLERANCE FACTOR

Glucose Tolerance Factor (GTF) isn't an index number, but a molecule best described as a 'chromium complex'. It's also the most biologically efficient way for elemental chromium to enter the system. With chromium as its core component, GTF contains niacin (vitamin B3), glyacine cysteine and glutamic acid. It is best taken as a supplement in brewer's yeast. But if you're prone to yeast infections, brewer's yeast should be avoided as a source of absorbable chromium.

AYURVEDA

An Indian system that dates back 5,000 years, Ayurveda combines the healing arts with philosophy and spiritual principles – Ayur means 'life', veda means 'science'. Several of the techniques and herbs in this book are ayurvedic, as a significant proportion of their remedies are relative to blood sugar imbalances and diabetes. Here, there is only space to scratch the Ayurvedic surface, but there are several books available that explain this fascinating health system in more detail.

SUPPLEMENTS
FOR DIABETES

Nutrient groups thought to help reverse insulin resistance and benefit diabetics are minerals, antioxidants, essential fatty acids and plant extracts. These are represented by some natural remedies and supplements that are pushing back the boundaries with evidence-based research. These natural remedies should, under no circumstances, be used as a replacement for insulin or other prescription drugs, merely as a complement. And they shouldn't be used without first seeking professional advice.

PYCNOGENOL

New research from the Institute of Pharmaceutical Chemistry at the University of Münster in Germany showed that Type II diabetes patients had lower blood sugar and healthier blood vessels after supplementing with French maritime pine tree bark extract, Pycnogenol. A study was carried out on patients aged 28–64 years who had mild type II diabetes and a BMI of between 22 and 34. The 18 men and 12 women were on a regular diet and exercise programme. The researchers reported that the patients were able to significantly lower glucose levels when they took 50–200 mg of the supplement.

Fish is a great source of vitamin B complex, which breaks down fats and carbohydrates and help the body to make use of insulin.

Antioxidant Pycnogenol is extracted from the bark of the Maritime pine that grows along the coast of southwest France. It has also been shown to improve cardiovascular problems prevailing in diabetics, as well as reduce high blood pressure, platelet aggregation, LDL-cholesterol and enhance circulation.

ALPHA-LIPOIC ACID (ALA)
Alpha-lipoic acid is a vitamin-like substance found in minute amounts in the body. It is also available in foods such as spinach, liver and brewer's yeast, but as it's hard to source in therapeutic amounts, it may be useful to take a supplement. ALA seems to offer all-round benefits to sufferers of diabetes: German researchers have found that ALA increases cellular uptake of glucose by 50 per cent. It appears to stimulate insulin activity, but reduces insulin resistance in diabetics. It is also a powerful anti-oxidant that has been used to treat diabetic neuropathy. In one study, daily doses of 600 mg ALA over three weeks were shown to reduce the symptoms of diabetic peripheral neuropathy.

FENUGREEK
This culinary spice has been used medicinally since the days of the pyramids. As regards the treatment of diabetes, the fenugreek seeds contain the two alkaloids trigonelline and coumarin which improve glucose tolerance. Regular ingestion has been shown to lead to a significant reduction in sugar in the urine, to improve cholesterol levels and to contribute to the body's successful management of blood sugar levels.

Whole fenugreek seeds can be baked into bread and cakes or, after soaking, eaten in muesli or cereal, while the powder can be suspended in water or juice and enjoyed as a drink. Bear in mind, though, that fenugreek has to be used in fairly large amounts – about three tablespoons a day – to have significant results. However, it is inexpensive and at nearly 30 per cent protein it has plenty of other benefits.

Fenugreek should not be taken during pregnancy, as it can set off uterine contractions.

GYMNEMA
The ancient Sanskrit name for this plant is Gur-mar, which literally means 'sweet blocker', as chewing its leaves leaves a residue on the tongue that cancels out any sugary tastes. This results in sweet foods tasting of not very much so that they rapidly lose their appeal.

Gymnema has been found to have a molecular make-up close to glucose, and when taken in tablet form will reduce blood-glucose levels and help regulate blood fat and cholesterol. Further to this, it has been shown to stimulate the regeneration of the pancreas' beta cells. These are vital to the body's insulin production and absorption, so any boost they receive can significantly reduce a sufferer's required insulin dosage.

VANADIUM
This trace element has been increasingly spoken of in recent years as a natural remedy for diabetes, but should be approached with extreme caution. Vadium moves sugar from the bloodstream into the muscle cells – it's used by body builders to build harder, denser muscles and turns up in muscle supplement foods. As a result, it functions much like insulin by regulating blood sugar swings. However, it has been found to accumulate in the muscles tissue and can result in a long-term toxic effect that appears to get worse with continued use. For this reason, it is impossible for us to recommend it at this stage until further tests have been done.

BITTER MELON
The juice of this lumpy green fruit is an ancient diabetic remedy of considerable hypoglycaemic worth. Sometimes referred to as 'plant insulin' due to a molecular structure very similar to bovine insulin, it will raise glucose tolerance and will protect the pancreas from free-radical damage, an accepted contributor to type I diabetes. Bitter melon can be sliced and eaten steamed or stir fried, while the dried essence can be brewed as tea, but the best way to take it is in its true bitter form - juiced. In some people, long-term ingestion may produce a toxic effect. ▶

FOR DIABETIC COMPLICATIONS

GINKO

Increases circulation, and allows more oxygen-rich red blood cells to the small blood vessels in the eyes that supply the retina. Can significantly reduce the likelihood of degenerative eye diseases associated with diabetes.

VITAMIN E

Greatly reduces the free radical damage that can lead to heart disease and nerve damage. Also reduces the build-up of fat that leads to clogged arteries.

ALPHA-LIPOIC ACID

A powerful antioxidant that combats diabetic neuropathy, the damaged nerve endings that can develop as a result of excessive blood sugar levels.

POLYPHENOLS AND FLAVENOIDS

These are plant-based compounds with powerful antioxidant properties that help to regulate blood sugar irregularities. Polyphenols and flavenoids are found in citrus fruit, brightly coloured berries and green vegetables. The best sources are: green tea, bilberries, ginko, milk thistle extract, buckwheat, hawthorn berry, red wine, and European coastal pine bark extract.

TURMERIC

Assists in the efficient management of cholesterol by lowering the level of serum cholesterol in the blood, while inhibiting its accumulation in the liver. Turmeric, which can be taken in capsules or as powder in drinks, also cuts the risk of arteries hardening by reducing platelet accumulation and lowering any risk of smooth muscle damage.

GARLIC

The real superstar of the natural remedy world – there's very little that garlic won't go some way towards fixing. Garlic is a proven hypoglycaemic, reducing glucose levels by imitating insulin in the liver and fooling the body into producing less, and going a long way to addressing any blood sugar imbalance. It also lowers LDL cholesterol while raising HDL cholesterol, and reduces blood pressure by thinning the blood. Eat as much garlic as you can.

GUGGUL

This Ayurvedic remedy is extracted from the resin of the mukul tree, a native plant of the Indian subcontinent, to produce gugulipids which have been shown to have a major impact on the treatment of heart disease and diabetes. What makes gugulipids so important is they are one of the very few compounds to regulate all fats in the body and reduce platelet stickiness. As a result, regular guggul ingestion lowers LDL cholesterol and triglycerides while raising HDL cholesterol, protects against clogging and hardening of the arteries, and protects the heart from damage by free radicals. Patients may have to take it regularly for two or three months before they notice any change.

KUTKI

Taken as a capsule, this herb boosts the digestive system to stimulate the pancreas to produce insulin secretion. It also promotes liver performance to regulate blood sugar stored in it as the glycogen that is vital for the body to cope with diabetes. ◼

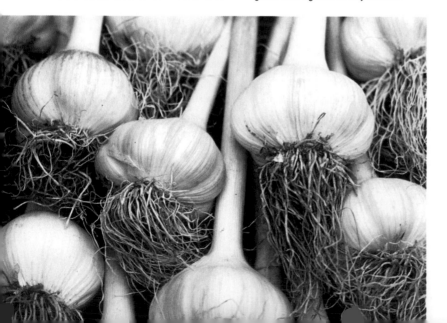

Garlic is full of health-giving properties: it regulates blood sugar, thins the blood and manages cholesterol levels.

VITAMINS AND MINERALS

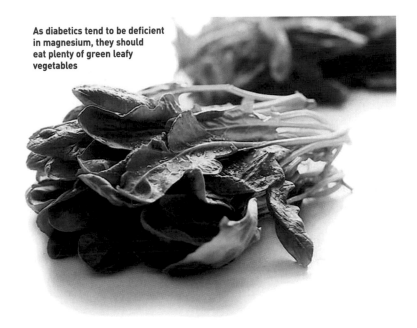

As diabetics tend to be deficient in magnesium, they should eat plenty of green leafy vegetables

The way modern food is farmed and processed often leaves a shortfall in vital vitamins and minerals. Getting enough of them is a crucial part of diabetes control, and these are the ones you cannot afford to go without.

CHROMIUM

What does it do?
Regulates the degree of glucose in the bloodstream, maintains a blood sugar balance, controls cholesterol levels, ensures efficient insulin function and can provoke insulin production in the pancreas.

Why do you need it?
Chromium deficiency is believed to contribute to people becoming diabetic later in life. A lack of chromium can cause blood sugar fluctuations, high cholesterol and may play a part in obesity. Prolonged physical and mental exertion will increase the need for chromium, while too much sugar in the diet will deplete the body's natural reserves. The typical Western diet is low in chromium, and it's especially needed by the young, old, pregnant, overweight and those who exercise.

Where can you find it?
Egg yolks, red wine, potato skins, broccoli, whole grains, black pepper and brewer's yeast.

Recommended daily dosage
30 mcg

MAGNESIUM

What does it do?
Improves both insulin resistance and blood sugar control. Also vital for a healthy heart and cardiovascular function, and will lower high blood pressure by reducing muscle tension in the artery walls.

Why do you need it?
It is estimated that 25 per cent of people with diabetes are deficient in magnesium and those with a low level in their diet or in their blood are far more likely to develop type II diabetes.

Where can you find it?
Brazil nuts, wheat germ, green leafy vegetables, whole grains – nearly all magnesium is lost from grain when it is milled. Refined sugar and carbohydrate will also have been virtually stripped on any magnesium content.

Recommended daily dosage
300 mg

VITAMIN B COMPLEX

What does it do?
Thiamine, pantothenic acid, niacin, pyridoxine and vitamin B12 are vital to break down fats and carbohydrates, and will assist the body in making use of insulin. Niacin lowers LDL cholesterol, triglycerides and fibrogen (a blood protein responsible for clot formation) and it is very important for maintaining blood sugar levels.

Why do you need it?
Without these vitamins you won't be regulating your blood sugar as efficiently as possible and insulin in your system – both natural and additional – will not be utilized effectively.

Where can you find it?
Significant amounts of niacin occur in peanuts, whole grains, brewer's yeast, sesame seeds, fish and meats.

Recommended daily dosage
80 mg

HOLISTIC THERAPIES

Although these complementary therapies won't cure diabetes, they can assist with blood flow and stress-level management, both of which are hugely important to diabetics.

TRANSCENDENTAL MEDITATION (TM)

TM is a wonderful, life-enriching therapy for relaxing and resting the mind and body. It involves silently and internally repeating a specific mantra, chosen specifically to suit your individual personality and psyche. The practice enables you to achieve a restful, yet alert state. Studies have shown that TM affects you physiologically as well as emotionally. Blood pressure, hypertension, anxiety, depression and insomnia all benefit. The beauty is that you can perform TM anywhere – commuters even practise it on the train – and it doesn't involve active movements, so is perfect for people whose mobility is impaired or who are experiencing pain.

MEDICAL QIGONG

Medical Qigong is a form of Chinese Energetic Medicine and is one of the four founding schools of Traditional Chinese Medicine. The phrase 'Qigong' is made of two words, 'Qi' and 'Gong'. Qi can be interpreted as life energy

Stress can send blood sugar levels soaring, so as a diabetic it's essential to find ways to relax.

or life force. The philosophy states that if a person is unwell, Qi is said to flow excessively or weakly through the body compared to when they are in good health. 'Gong' means cultivation, development or management. When Qi is properly cultivated a person remains in good mental, emotional and physical health. Although powerful on its own, when used in conjunction with other treatments, Medical Qigong accelerates healing.

Qigong therapy and prescriptions combine the use of breath work with individual physical movements, creative visualization, and perceptual intention. The primary goal is to purge toxic emotions from within the body's tissues, eliminate energetic stagnations, as well as strengthen and balance the internal organs and energetic fields. Medical Qigong practitioners either show patients how to do specific,

gentle exercises for themselves or perform management treatments for their patients. The International Institute of Medical Quigong says the discipline has positive, clinically recognized effects on weight management, bone strength and slow ageing, blood flow, blood pressure, heart function, kidney processes, eyesight and immune function.

ACUPUNCTURE

This is a complementary therapy that has particular applications for pain and neurological disorders, and for diabetics, acupuncture is very relevant.

"Given that diabetes is a chronic disease there is a range of things acupuncture can help with, particularly peripheral neuropathy," explains Professor Nicky Robinson, Professor of Complementary Medicine at Thames Valley University in the UK. "It can help

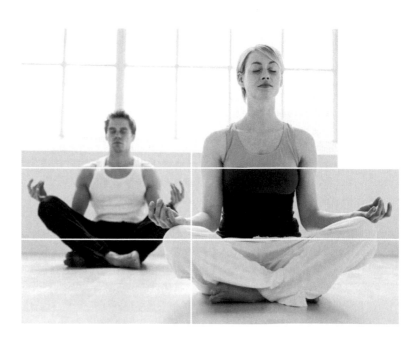

reduce pain, tingling and numbness and it can help with nerve supply to the bladder."

Acupuncture can't cure diabetes, but it can help relieve some of the side effects. According to the traditional Chinese philosophy on which the treatment is based, human health depends on the flow of Qi, which is channelled through meridians beneath the skins surface. Acupuncturists insert very fine needles into the skin where the energy flows, to try to stimulate the body's own healing response and restore balance.

"There has not been a lot of Western research done," admits Professor Robinson, 'but anecdotal evidence shows it may have a role to play in lowering blood glucose levels." Professor Robinson advises that acupuncture be used in conjunction with conventional medicine, and that if you begin any sort of complementary therapies, you should keep your doctor informed. When carried out by a trained acupuncturist, it could be a valuable addition to your diabetes care routine.

"Recently a large study showed there is a very low risk of serious adverse side effects," says Professor Robinson. "But I should emphasize that the acupuncturist must be a professionally qualified practitioner, who uses clean, single-use needles. For anyone suffering from leg ulceration there is a potential increased risk of infection."

A course of treatment normally lasts four to six weeks, then the patient is reassessed to check progress.

Massage
The main benefits of massage for a diabetic are for stress, digestion and the circulatory system. Most types of massage have a calming effect which in turn helps the digestive process. This is because in times of high stress adrenalin floods the body and inhibits food being processed and absorbed, which in turn causes blood sugar level to shoot up. Reducing your stress levels means the insulin is able to serve its intended purpose.

Releasing muscle tension can also encourage better circulation. Insulin-dependent diabetics should note that massage on injection sites can speed up insulin absorption and have a juice drink near to hand in case of a hypo (see page 32).

YOGA FOR HEALTH

Yoga has become immensely popular as more and more people discover the all-round benefits for mental and physical health.

Despite its origins thousands of years ago in India, yoga has just as much relevance to today's lifestyle – in fact some might argue it's more important now than ever before. Although most people often just think of the physical exercises, there are five principles to yoga: proper breathing, proper relaxation, a proper diet, meditation and proper exercise (hatha yoga). The five elements are designed to work together as a holistic system of mind and body therapy.

The exercise takes the form of asanas or postures which are designed to bring about a harmonious balance in the body. There are different styles of hatha yoga: Sivananda (gentler), Iyengar (focussing on postures), Vikram (performed at very high temperatures to make you sweat) and Ashtanga (more vigorous and producing immense internal heat). If you are practising one of the more energetic styles of hatha yoga, be alert for hypos.

No matter which style you choose, you'll derive many benefits from it.

Yoga helps reduce stress levels, increases fitness and promotes an active lifestyle, loosens up joints and aids mobility, stimulates the circulation and lowers blood pressure. By doing so, it can go a long way to preventing future diabetic complication.

Yoga cannot cure diabetes but it can help control glucose levels and ensure that your body is working at its optimum level. People who enjoy yoga also tend to opt for a healthier diet and lifestyle, and improve their self control, all of which are beneficial.

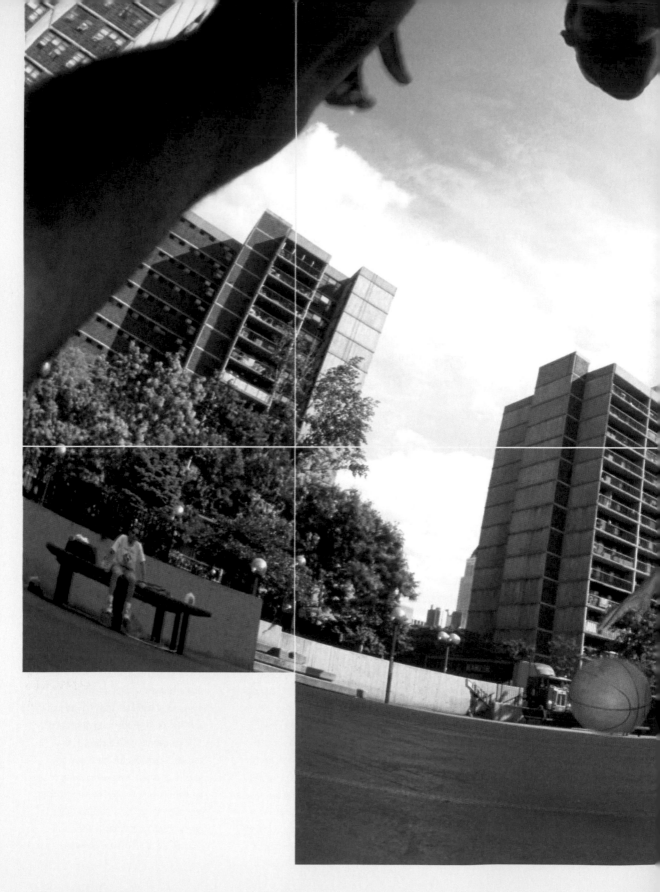

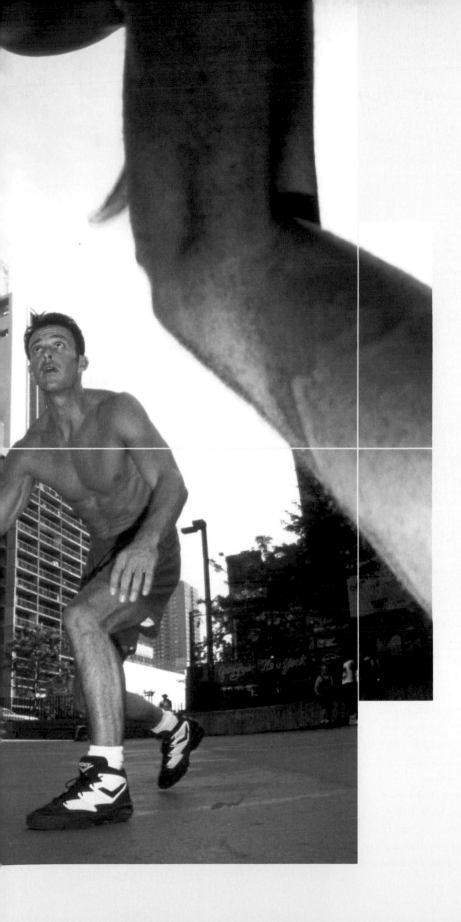

GET FIGHTING FIT

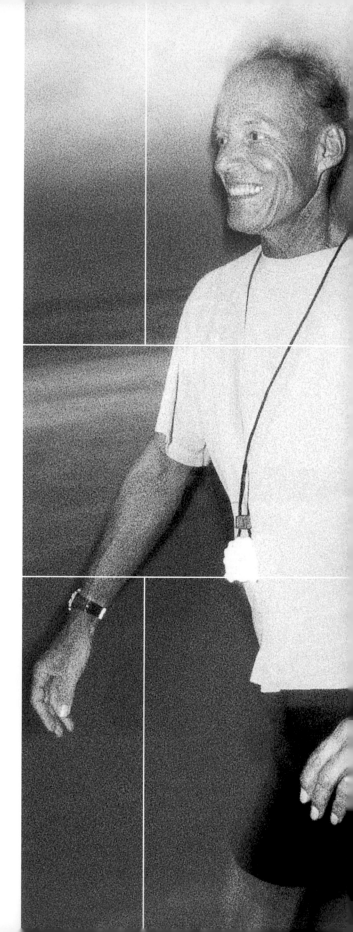

GET FIT TO FIGHT DIABETES

EVERYBODY CAN BENEFIT FROM EXERCISING REGULARLY BUT FOR DIABETICS, IT IS MORE OF A 'MUST' THAN A 'SHOULD'. REGULAR EXERCISE IS ONE OF THE MOST POWERFUL WEAPONS FOR CONTROLLING DIABETES AND LIVING A HEALTHY LIFE.

WE'VE ALREADY STRESSED THE importance of eating right in your fight against diabetes, however that's only half the story: getting and keeping fit is the absolutely vital other side of the coin.

Regular exercise is probably the best prescription any diabetic can follow for a number of reasons, the most obvious being those that also benefit non-diabetics: being fit makes you feel generally better, it allows you to do anything physical that bit more easily, it means you won't get tired so quickly, and it helps you to relax. The result is you're much more mentally alert and the risk of heart disease is greatly reduced, thanks in no small part to more efficient blood flow.

For a diabetic, regular exercise will also help enormously in keeping weight in check which is not so much an aesthetic consideration as a life-saving one. Maintaining a level of physical activity is particularly important to older, type II diabetics

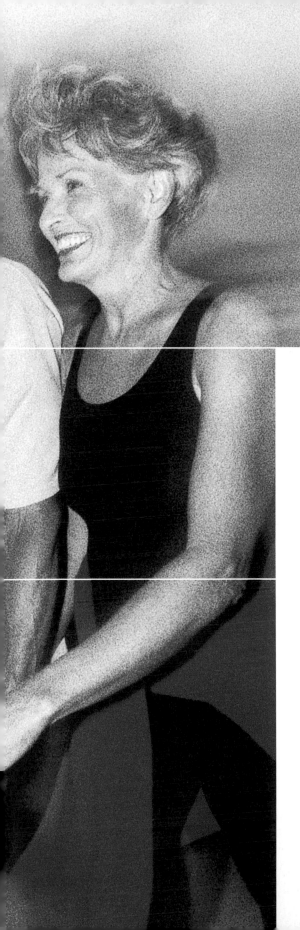

IF THE SHOE FITS

For anybody doing any form of exercise that involves running, walking or jumping, correctly fitting shoes are vital. But for a diabetic, it is more important than most. Because the onset of diabetes can lead to a condition known as 'diabetic neuropathy' or nerve damage in the hands and feet (see page 17), apparently minor injuries can go unnoticed and quickly become serious. So foot care and sock and shoe selection must be taken extra seriously.

■ Buy your shoes from a specialist running or sporting shop where they are sold for how they perform rather than just how they look.
■ Get your feet measured widthways as well as lengthways every time you buy a new pair of shoes.
■ Wear the socks you are going to wear for exercising when you try on the shoes.
■ Buy shoes in the afternoon not the morning – feet can swell by up to half a size during the course of the day.
■ Ask the assistant to check your gait – either running or walking – while you are trying the shoes on to make sure you get what is absolutely best for you.

as the metabolism may be slowing down. Keeping in shape greatly enhances cardiovascular efficiency – and how well the heart and lungs work has a direct bearing on the whole metabolism. This means that other vital organs such as the liver and the pancreas function far better. Regular exercise can assist in insulin and blood sugar management too. In China, research showed people with high blood sugar levels who engaged in moderate exercise were 40 per cent less likely to develop diabetes than their sedentary counterparts. And, most importantly for diabetics, regular exercise can boost glucose tolerance and reduce the need for insulin to be taken – drops in blood glucose ▶

levels of between 20 and 30 per cent after a single exercise session are not unusual.

The reason for this dramatic lowering of blood glucose levels is that regular exercising allows the body to use insulin in the most efficient way and to fulfil some of insulin's functions without actual recourse to it. Physical activity opens the pores on the muscle cell walls to allow the blood glucose that hard-working muscles require to be absorbed without the need for extra insulin to help the process. What insulin is present is used to the absolute maximum, and the muscles soak up enough glucose to stop levels in the blood getting dangerously high. To keep this process going, you should keep active throughout the day – it is one of the best things a diabetic can do. It should be stressed though, that any exercise programme should not be embarked

THE SPORTING LIFE

There is no reason whatsoever why any diabetic, provided they are fit enough and take a few simple precautions, shouldn't play practically any sport at practically any level. Indeed, five times Olympic gold medal winner Steve Redgrave – one of Great Britain's most successful athletes ever – is diabetic.

As well as being sure to rigidly adhere to the guidelines set out on page 88, be certain to make your instructor or coach aware that you are a diabetic and that he or she fully understands what to do should there be any problems. Also, inform your teammates of your condition, and reassure them there's nothing to worry about. A few sports governing bodies have regulations that prevent insulin-injecting diabetics from joining and therefore competing on an official level, and while any registered coach should be aware of any such rules, Diabetes UK (see page 156) will have further information about these sporting bodies and their regulations.

GIVE YOURSELF TIME

To get the most benefit out of your exercise regime from the start, you should work out three times a week and, initially, allow an hour per session. That means 10 minutes to warm up, 10 minutes to warm down and 40 minutes for exercising. Duration and/or frequency should increase as you progress, but this is the bare minimum of usefulness for beginners.

upon without first consulting your doctor or diabetes care team, as strenuous activity for insulin-dependent diabetics or for those who are seriously overweight could be potentially harmful.

This doesn't mean that you can't exercise, it simply means you should get the advice of a qualified diabetes practitioner as to the best type of exercise for you and how to adjust your medication accordingly, either prior to and/or after your training session. Nor does it mean that some sort of mild physical activity – walking up stairs instead of taking the lift, getting off the bus a stop earlier, or taking a daily stroll around the block – shouldn't become part of your new, healthy regime. Just don't jump straight into two hours a day in the gym or running a marathon. It's not uncommon for insulin-dependent diabetics to have their dosages reduced in conjunction with regular exercise schedules but this should never be contemplated without first consulting your doctor.

Starting out

The thing is to be sensible about how you exercise, especially when you're starting out. Even exercising a little bit more than you do now is a good thing and to do any exercise as opposed to none at all is infinitely better. Start with what you know you can fit in to your life and build up from there as you start to get into

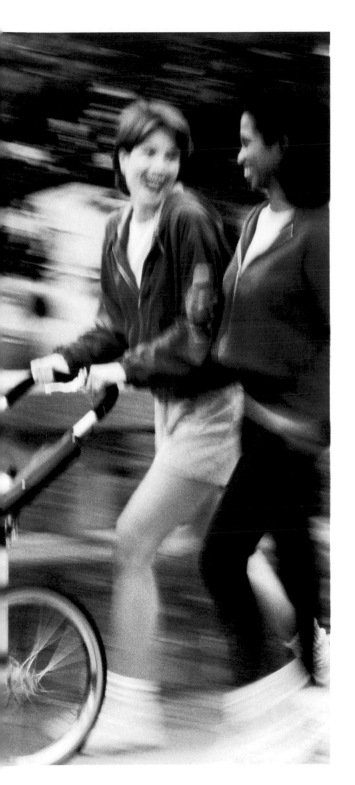

ACTIVITY CALORIE COUNTER

The following table can only be an approximation, as how many calories you burn during an hour's worth of activity depends entirely on how much effort you put into it! However, this table will give you an idea of how various activities compare to each other, and how as a result you should adjust your pre-exercise calorie intake.

ACTIVITY	CALORIES BURNT
SQUASH	800 calories
SWIMMING	400/700 calories
JOGGING 12 km/h (8 mph)	600 calories
CYCLING 15 km/h (10 mph)	500 calories
AEROBICS (mid level)	500 calories
CIRCUIT TRAINING	450 calories
JOGGING 10 km/h (6 mph)	450 calories
BASKETBALL	450 calories
POWER WALKING	450 calories
NETBALL	400 calories
FOOTBALL	360 calories
BADMINTON	350 calories
WALKING	300 calories
YOGA	300 calories

it, and pick a form of exercise that won't do you any damage. In general, an aerobic or cardio-vascular workout will be of most use for those with diabetes, but there are many different types and it will be vital to choose the one most suitable for you, and even more importantly one that you enjoy!

According to Diabetes UK, walking briskly for 30 minutes five times a week has been nationally adopted as the minimum requirement for healthy benefits. Thirty minutes spread over the day is equally beneficial, and activity within your ▶

THE GOLDEN RULES OF WORKING OUT SAFELY

■ Choose an activity suitable both for your level of fitness and the time available. While you should be prepared to stretch yourself, don't overdo it in the beginning.

■ Discuss any proposed exercise schedule with your doctor before embarking on it.

■ Check your blood glucose level before and after your workout, and keep records.

■ Don't make any adjustments to your insulin intake without prior consultation with your doctor.

■ Eat a carbohydrate snack with roughly the same calories as you are about to expend (see table page 87). If you need to lose weight, consume less calories than you burn.

■ Have glucose drinks or tablets nearby. Wear a clearly visible diabetic identity bracelet or tag, and if road running or cross-country running, make sure you tell somebody where you are going and carry a mobile phone or a card with your contact details.

■ Be aware of hypos and insulin irregularity warning signs – if you feel faint, dizzy or confused, stop working out straight away, check your blood sugar level if you can and drink some fruit juice or a glucose drink if necessary.

■ Drink plenty of water before, during and after your workout, as dehydration can raise blood sugar levels.

■ Do not exercise if tests reveal you have high blood sugar levels or ketones in your urine. It means you don't have enough insulin in your system to make use of the glucose your liver will produce during exercise, so your levels will spike.

daily routine can also burn calories and improve metabolic function, such as your body's response to insulin. Brisk or 'power' walking is ideal for the elderly or the arthritic as its impact is much lower than running and so will put far less stress on the knees and ankles. Riding a stationary bike or using an airwalker is another excellent low-impact form of aerobic exercise. Swimming is a fantastic full-body workout with hardly any wear and tear on the joints, and can be useful to almost everybody.

Jogging or cycling are ideal for younger people or those less susceptible to joint pains, as are sports such as squash, basketball or football. (Resistance or weight training by itself is less useful for diabetics, as its primary function is to build muscle mass rather than increase cardiovascular efficiency or to burn fat.) The important thing to remember when doing sport is to take on extra calories beforehand. How much will depend on how vigorous the sport is – but it is vital for a diabetic to have something in the bank before starting the activity. Even then, as an added precaution to any adverse insulin reaction, it is advisable to have fruit juice or a glucose drink readily available while exercising.

And it is a good idea to remember that your body will continue to use extra energy to replenish body stores even after an activity has ended so extra carbohydrates may be needed directly after the activity, and at snack and meal times. The type of snacks you take will depend on what is suitable and convenient for the activity you are doing.

Finally, whatever the exercise, if you start a work-out programme you should monitor your blood sugars before and after every session and keep records. This is important to establish what that particular activity actually does to your sugar levels and to make you aware of any possibly dangerous dips or spikes. ◙

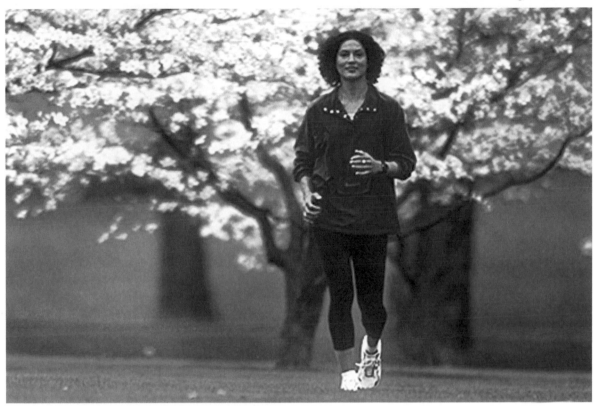

WHICH WORKOUT IS FOR YOU?

Every activity will affect your body differently so make sure you choose the right one for you.

ACTIVITY: Walking
GOOD FOR: More or less everybody, especially those just starting out exercising and older participants
NOT SO GOOD FOR: N/A

ACTIVITY: Power walking
GOOD FOR: Beginners who want a more challenging workout
NOT SO GOOD FOR: The very overweight

ACTIVITY: Jogging
GOOD FOR: Fitter, more robust participants
NOT SO GOOD FOR: Those with joint or bone trouble

ACTIVITY: Aerobics
GOOD FOR: Although there are classes at different levels, they can be daunting for the beginner

NOT SO GOOD FOR: Those with joint or bone trouble or heart problems

ACTIVITY: Weight lifting
GOOD FOR: N/A
NOT SO GOOD FOR: Because it's resistance rather than cardiovascular training, it won't help much for either weight loss or fighting diabetes

ACTIVITY: Swimming
GOOD FOR: Everybody, even those who have difficulty walking can swim for exercise
NOT SO GOOD FOR: N/A

ACTIVITY: Sport (netball, basketball football etc)
GOOD FOR: The already physically fit who have time to spare
NOT SO GOOD FOR: The demands of organized sports might be too much for those just starting out

GET FIT WITH AN AEROBIC WORKOUT

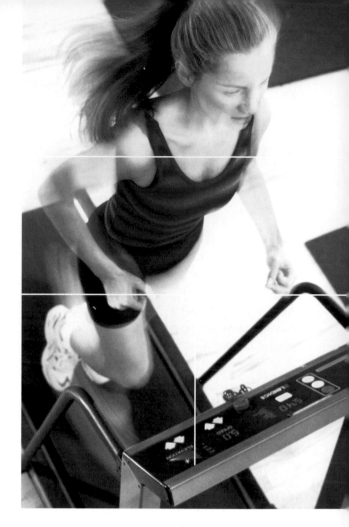

A PROPER WARM-UP AND COOL-DOWN ARE VITAL PARTS OF ANY EXERCISE SESSION. ANY TIME YOU DO ANY ACTIVITY THAT IS SIGNIFICANTLY HARDER THAN YOUR NORMAL EVERYDAY LIVING, YOU NEED TO PREPARE YOUR BODY FOR THE CHALLENGES IT IS ABOUT TO FACE, AND EASE IT BACK DOWN TO NORMAL AFTERWARDS. REMEMBER, NONE OF THIS COUNTS AS PART OF YOUR ACTUAL EXERCISE SESSION – IT IS EXTRA.

WARMING UP

Loosen up Spend five minutes walking around and gently loosening your joints and muscles so they don't pull. Make circles in the air with your arms, wrists, hips and ankles, shrug your shoulders, swing your legs back and forth and bend and straighten your knees. Feel your range of motion gently increase, but never force yourself to the limits.

Raise your heart rate For the next 5–10 minutes, gradually increase your exercise pace from very, very easy to just slightly harder than the pace you want to maintain for the main part of your session. (So, if you're out for a run start with walking, then easy jogging, then slow running, then your 'training' pace, then just a shade faster.)

Re-stretch Finally, spend a minute or two gently and briefly stretching the muscles you will be exercising. Don't force the stretch at all – you're not trying to increase your flexibility. Hold each stretch for 10–15 seconds.

COOLING DOWN

Ease back At the end of your training, spend five minutes gradually reducing your speed until you're working very easily once again.

Get warm You'll probably be hot and sweaty after exercise, but you'll soon get cold. Stay warm by putting on extra clothing and going indoors.

Drink Your body may also be slightly dehydrated after exercise, so try to have a good drink (a pint of water) soon after you stop.

Stretch Muscles and tendons can stiffen up after exercise so keep them limber and injury-free by spending 10-15 minutes stretching all your major muscle groups. Pay particular attention to the muscles that worked the most during, ie legs if you cycled, and back and shoulders if you swam. Take each stretch as far as comfortable, and hold for 30–60 seconds without bouncing or tensing any muscles. ◼

FEEL THE BURN

Aerobic exercise is a guaranteed fat burner, but it doesn't have to be a killer workout as well. You can start off as gently as you like and still feel the burn. Indeed, it's not unusual for absolute beginners to begin by simply sitting in a chair, doing the arm actions and kicking their legs. Remember, doing any more exercise than you do already is going to have a positive effect. The aerobic exercises outlined in this section are very basic and can be carried out as easily as you like. Endurance will vary depending on how fit you are when you are doing them,

and it's best to go for repetitions rather than timing. Between 10 and 20 steps with each leg is ideal and you can increase the pace of the routine from there. Start slowly and speed up as you go along and get fully warmed up before you up the pace. These exercises are good for both men and women, and although they're shown with a step, practise without one until you are doing 20 or so reps without any strain as to step up is considerably more difficult. Don't forget, in an aerobic workout there is no resting between reps!

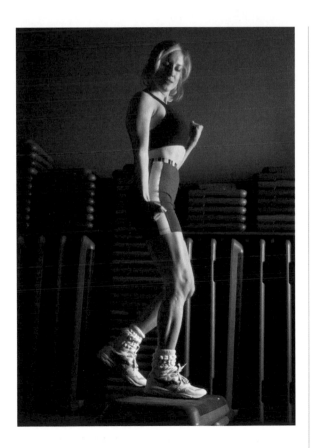

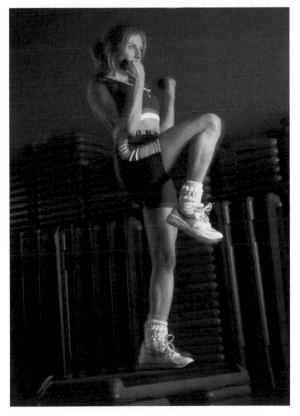

Step up with your right foot, bring your left foot up level with it and take your weight. It's vital you bring the left foot up to take some weight in order to complete a step.

Raise your right knee as high as you can, and bend you arms at the elbow. Step down with your right foot. Repeat, leading with your left foot. ▶

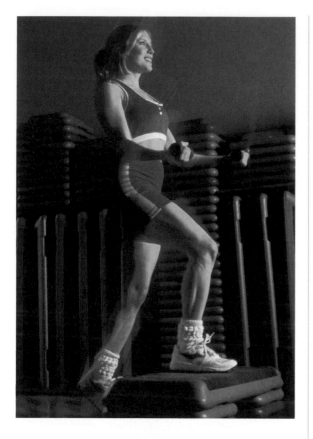 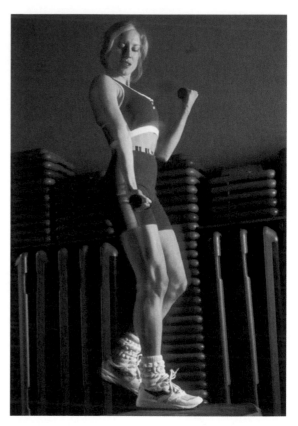

Step up with your right foot as before and follow with your left foot. This time, as you step down, bring your elbows behind you until your fists are past your waist.

Step up with your right foot and bring your left foot up to meet it. Do alternate arm curls, keeping your elbows close to your body.

HOW EXERCISE WORKS

1 When you begin to exercise at a moderate intensity, you increase the demands on your muscles.

2 To meet these demands your muscles need more fuel. Even at low 'fat-burning' intensities, the body still needs sugar to fuel the brain and nervous system, and convert fat to energy in muscles.

3 Converting this fuel to energy, requires oxygen, so the heart begins to beat faster and your breathing increases to provide more oxygen to the muscles.

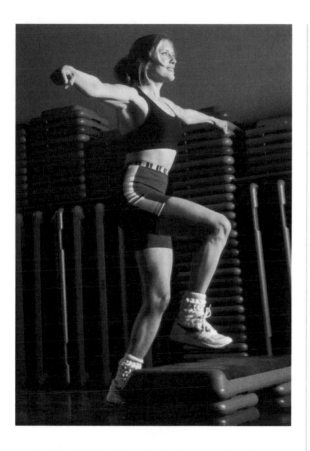

Step up with your right foot and bring your left foot. As you step back raise your arms out straight at the shoulders, returning them to your sides as you finish the step.

SAFETY FIRST

■ Warm up thoroughly before starting out (see page 90).

■ Whether you're a beginner or advanced, don't forget to eat about half an hour before starting your workout.

■ Drink plenty of fluids before, during and after exercising.

■ Remember to take your blood sugar readings before and after exercising, and during if you start to feel a hypo coming on.

■ Don't torture yourself – this isn't boot camp. If you start to feel wobbly for any reason, stop, sit down and take a blood sugar reading. You will do yourself lasting damage if you carry on exercising when your body cannot cope with it.

4 Because exercise puts a strain on the body, it responds by trying to work as efficiently as possible. The most easily available fuel for exercise is blood sugar.

5 Diabetics tend to have unusually high levels of blood sugar, and this will be used as the first choice fuel source during exercise.

6 When blood sugar runs out, the liver releases glycogen to stabilize blood sugar and feed the nervous system and the muscles use muscle glycogen and fat as fuel. ◻

WALK YOUR WAY TO GOOD HEALTH

EXERCISE DOESN'T HAVE TO BE HI-TECH OR HI-IMPACT OR EVEN HI-ENERGY. SOMETIMES THE SIMPLEST ROUTINE CAN HAVE THE SAME BENEFICIAL EFFECT, AND ROUTINES DON'T COME SIMPLER THAN WALKING.

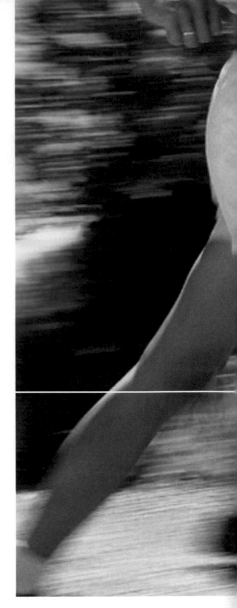

Perhaps you've previously been unable to exercise rigorously due to health, disability or age, but have now been advised, as a diagnosed diabetic, to incorporate exercise into your lifestyle. Or, you have simply been intimidated by the thought of joining a gym or going jogging. If so, try walking.

As a diabetic, even a small increase in your physical activity is desirable as exercise plays a huge part in controlling your blood glucose levels, protecting your heart and reducing the risk of diabetes-related complications such as nerve or eye damage. Walking around the home or office can help enormously as can getting off the bus a stop earlier, using the toilets on the next floor or leaving the car at home when you nip down to the local shops. However, although any exercise is better than none, this will be fairly unquantifiable and the way to get much greater benefit from walking is to draw up a plan with achievable and escalating goals. That way you can monitor your progress to fitness and better health.

The first thing you need to do is buy a pedometer – any good sports shop should sell them – a device not much bigger than a wristwatch that straps to one of your ankles and records the number of steps you take. By wearing this, you can calculate your walking baseline, which is how many steps you take per day taken as an average over three days. Your target figure, to be reached in two to three weeks' time, is 10,000 steps per day.

To work out your daily quota, subtract your baseline figure from 10,000 and divide that number by however many days you think it will take you to reach 10,000 steps. The fitter among you will be dividing by 14 (two weeks), while those at the other end of the scale will divide it by 21 (three weeks). The answer is the number of steps you must add on to your walking every day to reach the target figure. Wear your pedometer every day to measure these individual targets and keep track of how you are doing by keeping a walking log.

When approached like this, even gentle exercise such as walking can have a dramatic effect on your energy levels, blood glucose control, weight-loss plan and all round fitness. Walking 10,000 steps a day has been proved to be sufficient aerobic exercise to significantly help protect you against a number of different illnesses, of which diabetes is only one – others include heart disease, osteoporosis and some cancers. Also, as it can incorporated into your daily life, it is much easier for people to achieve walking 10,000 steps a day than it might be to go to the gym for half an hour.

Once you have achieved the 10,000

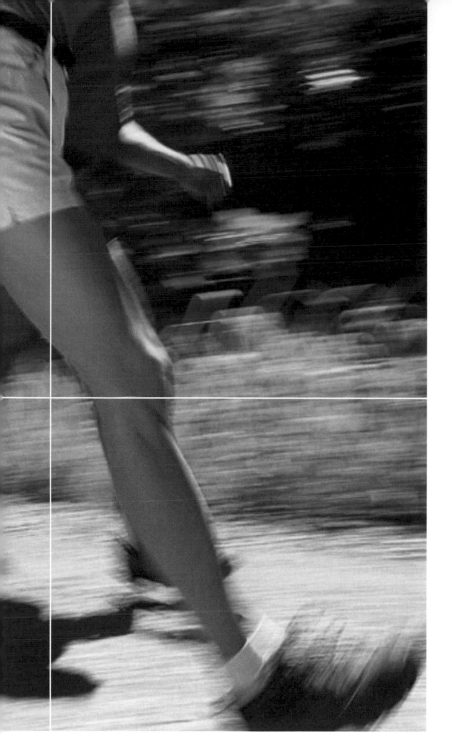

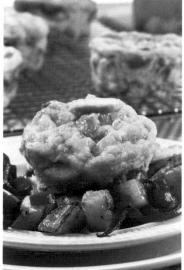

DON'T FORGET

- Eat something 30 minutes before you start your walk.
- Check your blood glucose level before and after every walk to make sure you are aware of any dangerous dips.
- Walk on your programme at least every other day.
- Get into a routine by walking at the same time each day.

steps-per-day target, there are several advanced walking alternatives. Interval walking involves walking a set time (one or two minutes) or set number of steps at a very fast pace, followed by the same time/number at a much slower 'recovery'. Hill walking requires considerably more effort and so gives a much greater workout, while power walking – fast with vigorous upper body movement – is a guaranteed calorie burner. If you have a dog, take it with you and encourage it to set a brisk pace, even break into a trot from time to time. And finally, control your pace and timing by listening to different tempos and styles of music while you walk. While this can help alleviating boredom, be careful of what's going on around you when you are exercising wearing headphones.

CUT DOWN THAT WAISTLINE... CUT DOWN THOSE HEALTH RISKS!

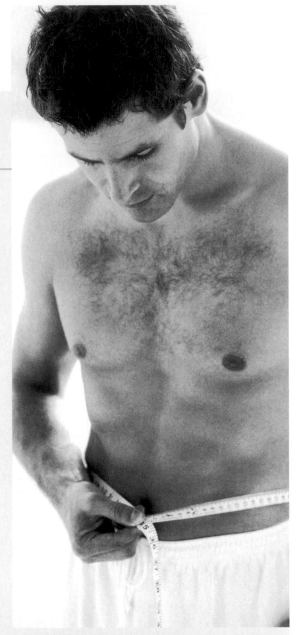

Lose the spare tyre, and not only will you look much better, you'll also have taken a major step towards living longer, as one of the most effective ways to fight diabetes is to banish your belly for ever.

Getting rid of that extra weight from your waistline is guaranteed to draw compliments, but this new slimline, sexy you will be working just as hard at saving your life. Recent research has demonstrated that the degree of abdominal fat a person has is directly related to their general health, notably heart disease and other cardio-vascular problems. The same research showed this to be particularly applicable as regards diabetes: for women of average height, those with a waist measurement greater than 90 cms (36 in) were five times more likely to develop diabetes than those with waistlines less than 70 cms (28 in). In the case of men, a measurement of more than 100 cms (40 in) meant a similar risk.

Unlike the fat on the rest of your body, belly fat is far more likely to release fatty acids into the liver, which can get broken down into ketones and maybe result in acid blood. Or, more crucially for diabetics, a super-sized tummy can interfere with blood sugar management as it can lead to excessive amounts of insulin and cholesterol in the bloodstream. Furthermore, there seems to be a definite link between abdominal fat and insulin resistance. As the term implies, this means that the cells no longer respond to insulin facilitating their absorbing blood sugar as efficiently as they should, leaving a glut of sugar in the bloodstream which can swiftly reach an dangerously high level. Should this condition continue – ie you refuse to lose that gut – it can result in the pancreas shutting down its insulin production, because the body appears to have no use for it, directly causing diabetes.

Thus it is absolutely vital for diagnosed diabetics, or those who believe they might be at risk, to keep that belly in check, and the best way to do that is with a combination of eating well and exercising right. The former is all explained in *The Food Factor* section starting on page 100 and to get you started with the latter, in conjunction with *Men's Health* magazine, we've put together a series of exercises that will work those abs to make you look as fit as you'll feel.

As with the aerobic exercises shown on pages 91-3, these can be done to equal effect by both men and women. Warming up beforehand is mandatory and the intensity of workout should be stepped up as you progress.

TRIM YOUR
WAISTLINE

THE ONLY WAY TO PERMANENTLY AND SAFELY REDUCE AND FIRM UP YOUR ABDOMEN
IS WITH A COMBINATION OF DIET AND EXERCISE. IT'S TIME TO GET PHYSICAL!

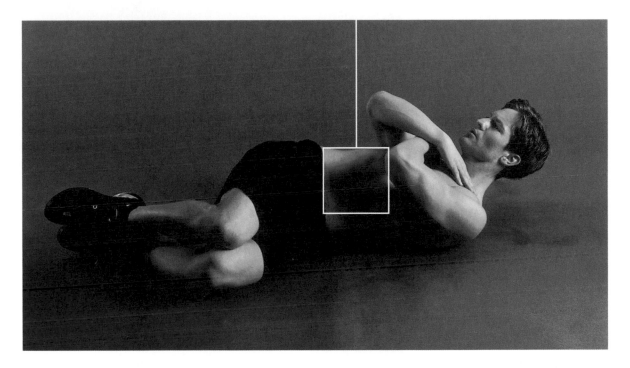

MOST PEOPLE WOULD LIKE THE KIND
of fat, firm tummy that turns heads on the beach.
A healthy eating plan (see page 122) is a good
start but to really get toned and stay in shape
you need to work out on a regular basis.

Don't worry though, the series of exercises
on the following pages, devised for us by
Men's Health magazine, can be used both by
those starting out and the very fit. Take the
exercise routine at your own pace and always
listen to the messages your body gives you.

THE PROGRAMME

Do the complete programme two or three times
a week for four weeks. Do a set of each exercise
in the first week, then two as a circuit in
subsequent weeks. A circuit is a set of each
exercise, catch your breath, then repeat. ▶

> Although we have used a man to demonstrate this
> series, like the exercises on the previous pages,
> they are equally suitable for women.

EXERCISE	ONE CIRCUIT	TWO CIRCUITS
Thin tummy	5 repetitions/3-second holds	5 repetitions/3-second holds
Curl up	5-10 repetitions	7 repetitions per circuit
Bridge	5 repetitions/3-second holds	5 repetitions/3-second holds
Thin tummy squeeze	5 repetitions/3-second holds	5 repetitions/3-second holds

STARFILE

STEVE REDGRAVE

"I went training one day and came home with a tremendous thirst – I first tried drinking one pint of water, then two pints and this was followed by a couple more but nothing was touching the thirst. At this stage I knew that something was wrong. My first thought when I was told it was diabetes was that my rowing career was at an end, but I spoke to my doctor and my specialist and both said I should be aware that the path to success was possible but not going to be easy. Really, there is very little known about endurance sports and diabetes so it's been a steep learning curve for all of us.

"Many people are unaware that they have diabetes or do not manage their diabetes effectively – at first I went into a denial phase as I did not want to accept that it was happening to me and I took as little insulin as possible. Now, as a type II diabetic injecting insulin, I test six or seven times a day and try and use my status to project a positive message and get people to think about the issues associated with testing."

EXERCISES
BEGINNER LEVEL

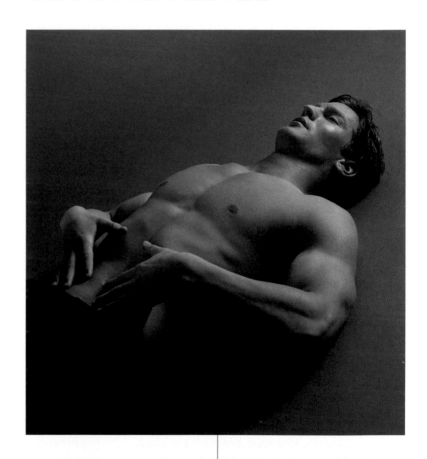

THIN TUMMY

Set-up: Lie on your back, knees bent, feet flat. Place both hands below your belt line with fingers pointed down and thumbs just below the rib cage.
Execution: Contract your lower abdominal muscles, to 'thin' your tummy between your belly button and groin and leave your upper abdominal muscles hollowed not pushed out. Hold for three seconds, relax, take a couple of deep breaths and repeat.

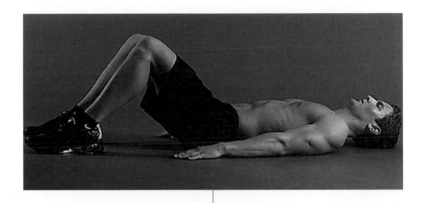

CURL UP

Set-up: Lie on your back with your feet flat on the floor and knees bent at a 90° angle. Your arms should be straight out on the floor beside you.
Execution: Supporting yourself with your arms – but not using them to push yourself up – raise your upper torso from the floor as far as you can, in a continuous controlled movement without jerking. Lower yourself back down just as smoothly, relax, take a couple of deep breaths and repeat.

SEATED THIN TUMMY & CHEEK SQUEEZE

Set-up: Sit on a chair or bench with your knees and feet together, your chest up and your back straight. Place both hands on your abdomen to assume the 'Thin Tummy' position described far left.
Execution: Contract your lower abdominal muscles, as in 'Thin Tummy', and at the same time clench your buttocks to raise yourself up in your seat – this action will intensify the work being done by the abdominal muscles. Hold for three seconds and relax both sets of muscles, breathe deeply and repeat. ◧

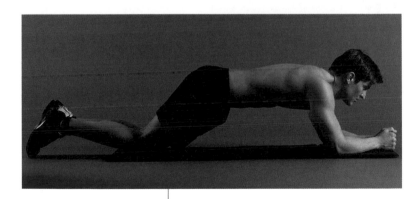

THE BRIDGE

Set-up: Kneel on the floor supporting your upper body on your forearms.
Execution: With your weight shifted to your toes, raise your knees from the floor to allow your back and legs to form a straight line at an angle to rather than parallel with the floor. Hold for three seconds and relax back on to your knees to take a couple of deep breaths before repeating.

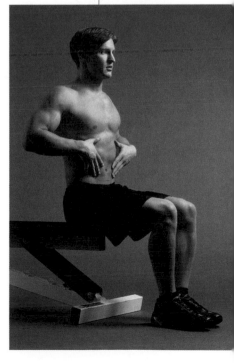

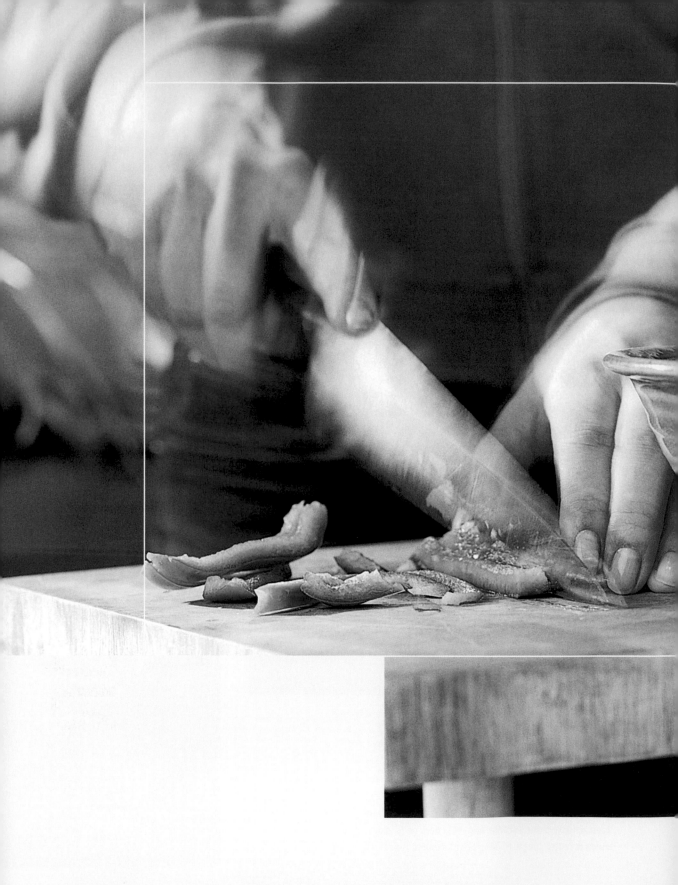

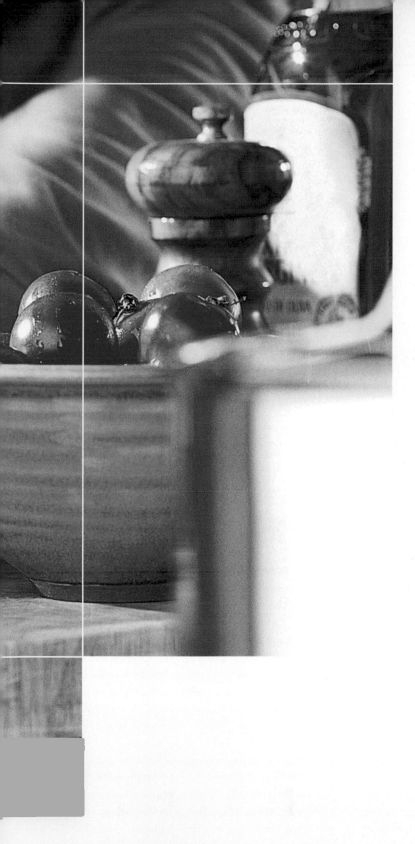

THE FOOD FACTOR

EATING RIGHT

AS WHAT YOU EAT PLAYS SUCH A HUGE PART IN BLOOD SUGAR AND CHOLESTEROL LEVELS, FOOD IS THE SINGLE MOST IMPORTANT FACTOR IN CONTROLLING DIABETES. BUT THERE'S NO REASON AT ALL WHY 'HEALTHY' CAN'T ALSO MEAN 'DELICIOUS' AND 'DESIRABLE'.

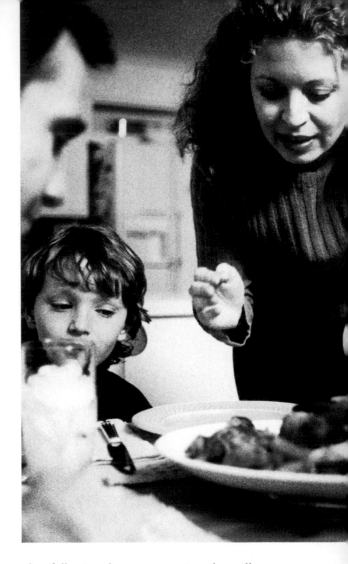

LIKE SO MUCH THAT CONCERNS people with diabetes, food is just a matter of taking something that ought to apply to everybody – eating right – and giving it a little extra thought and concentration. In other words, while a healthy eating plan is important for everybody, for a diabetic it can be absolutely crucial.

However, and this is the most exciting thing to remember, eating to control diabetes needn't be some sort of culinary purgatory in which you exist on lentils and broccoli, and every meal becomes something to be endured rather than enjoyed. Indeed, a quick thumb through our recipe section beginning (see pages 120–55) shows just how delicious and attractive healthy eating for diabetics can be. A diabetic's diet doesn't have to be dull if it uses natural ingredients and lateral thinking. It's all about being sensible and making sure you keep the right balance.

Firstly though, it's important to remember

that following the correct eating plan will not 'cure' your diabetes, nor will it remove your need for insulin. But what it can do is go a long way towards reducing your risk of attacks, possibly allow you to cut back on insulin doses – although talk to your doctor before you attempt this – and allow you to live a longer and more comfortable life. Also, the twin benefits of mental alertness and physical fitness that come with a healthy diet should be reason enough for anybody to adopt one, diabetic or not!

The official line as regards diabetic eating plans has evolved hugely in the last couple of decades as so much more is learned about the make-up of what we eat and how it works within our bodies. Previous thinking was that a diabetic should cut out all carbohydrates and seek to gain their calorific intake – needed for energy – from

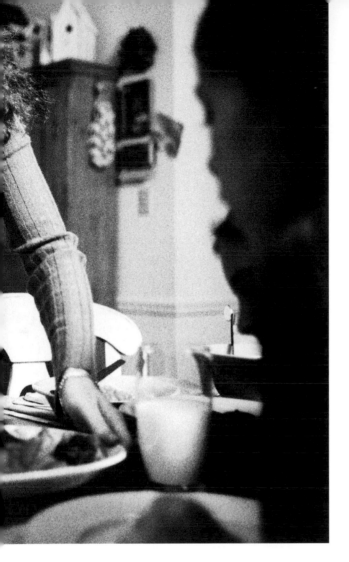

SHOULD YOU EAT SUGAR?

It's more a question of 'Can you eat sugar?', and the answer is yes, but with enormous reservations. In other words, sensible amounts of refined sugar can be enjoyed in limited quantities provided you are very careful. The problem with sugar is the speed at which it gets into your system, causing a dangerous peak in blood glucose. But this only happens when it is taken by itself without other carbohydrates – canned fizzy drinks are notorious offenders. To incorporate sugar into your healthy eating plan, it's vital you only take it as part of another food to block that fast-acting effect, and preferably at the end of a meal, when other food will already be in your stomach to cushion it. For an overall weight-management plan, make sure you count sugar instead of other carbohydrate foods not as well as, and be very careful that you know what you're eating. Check the ingredients on food packaging and bear in mind that such terms as lactose, fructose, sucrose, glucose, maltose, honey, molasses or corn syrup are all just different names for sugar.

protein and fat, a bit like the Atkins Diet. But this approach was oblivious to how excess protein increases the possibility of kidney problems, something diabetics can be more prone to, and that the amount of fat contained in meat and dairy products was always going to lead to weight gain, one of the prime causes of type II diabetes.

These days diabetes-controlling eating plans differentiate between the different types of carbohydrates and fats, creating a varied diet that's far more effective at balancing blood sugar levels. With this increased understanding of how what you eat works, it's even possible to enjoy the occasional sinfully sugary dessert without doing yourself any harm.

Sugar and fat are pretty much the bad guys when it comes to eating to control diabetes, and for good reason too. Although sugar contains

glucose that is vital for the body and brain to function, and sugar itself is an energy-providing carbohydrate, refined sugar – as found in packaged white sugar or in sweets, fizzy drinks, cakes or biscuits – is sucrose and has no nutritional benefits whatsoever. It provides completely empty calories. Worse than that, though, it is absorbed almost instantly into the bloodstream, so if consumed in large quantities and/or on an empty stomach, it can cause a dangerous leap in blood glucose levels.

Now that more is understood about how carbohydrates work, the modern approach to sugar in a diabetic eating plan is that it can be enjoyed in moderation but only as part of something else. To make this simple carbohydrate behave more like one of its complex cousins (see page 105 it needs to be mixed with other foods ▶

– preferably something fibrous – or consumed at the end of a meal to make sure the ballast is there to slow its absorption into the bloodstream. That is why sugary drinks or very sweet tea or coffee should remain off limits.

Fat has been greatly misunderstood. Beyond its obvious calorific value, fat is actually vital to how the body functions: it maintains cell wall production; carries the fat-soluble vitamins A, D, E and K through the bloodstream; and provides a lot of the flavour in meat and poultry. On the downside, though, too much fat is a weight problem waiting to happen and that is far more serious for a diabetic. Beyond that, it can lead to deposits called atheroma in the arteries, which will eventually harden reducing the internal size of the artery and therefore the blood flow levels within – it's these hardened deposits that break off to form the basis of blood clots.

However, modern research has shown it is a matter of what kind of fat you are eating as there are good and bad fats (see right), just as there is harmful and safe cholesterol. Saturated fats are the harmful fats that raise cholesterol levels in the arteries and cause a thickening, stickiness of the blood, greatly increasing the likelihood of heart disease. Monosaturated and polyunsaturated fats, on the other hand, are far more desirable. Indeed the former (found in olive oil) actually lowers the levels of cholesterol that does you harm, while the latter (in fish oils, sunflower and corn oils) lowers cholesterol levels all round. So rather than look to cut fat out of your diet all together, you could be doing more to maintain your general health levels and to fight diabetes by consuming the right type of fat.

As part of any diabetic or weight-loss eating plan though, it's worth remembering that it's

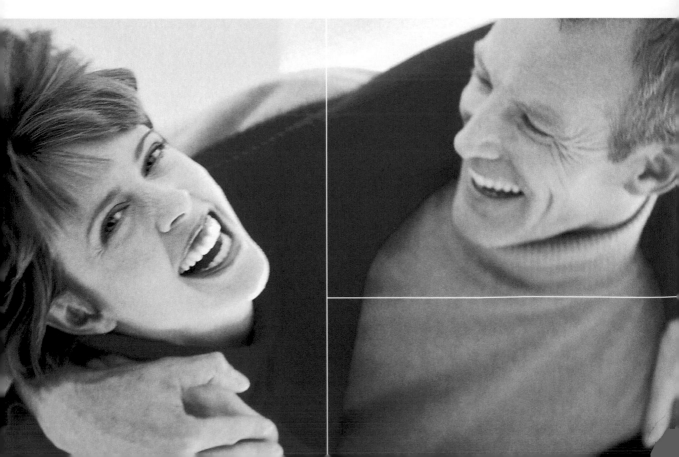

better to boil or steam food than fry it and better to shallow fry than deep fry. If you deep fry, drain the food on kitchen paper before serving to absorb as much surplus fat as possible.

Proteins are vital for cell repair and growth, but many adults eat far more than is needed. The only real risk of too much protein in itself is to a diabetic's kidneys, but some protein is much more advisable than others. Vegetable or plant-based protein, as found in beans and nuts, is far less risky than animal protein found in meat and dairy foods, because it contains less saturated fat.

Carbohydrates are another misunderstood part of most people's diet. They include a broad range of sugars, starches and fibres, are a major source of calories and fall into two categories: simple and complex. The first, sugar, is refined, and as discussed will deliver glucose quickly into the bloodstream. The complex carbohydrates, such as pulses, cereal, wholemeal bread and potatoes, contain starch and fibre as well as glucose, all of which slow down the absorption of glucose by blocking its passage (see panel page 108). Complex carbohydrates are much safer for the diabetic to take on as they avoid the blood sugar spikes that might be brought on by simple carbohydrates, and the fibre aids digestion by moving food through the system quicker.

As to the question of how much, if any, complex carbohydrates should figure in a healthy eating plan, diabetics are not advised to give them up completely as fibre is an important part of your diet. Foods high in starch – potatoes, pasta, rice, yams – are not recommended for type II diabetics as weight is more of an issue for those people and it's easy to overload on starch and so take on board extra calories. The safest carbohydrates for diabetics to eat are the ones that break down and release their glucose the slowest and will, therefore, have the least dramatic effect on blood sugar levels. But if you have a carbohydrate allowance set by your ▶

GOOD FAT, BAD FAT

Some fat is essential to keep the body functioning properly, but too much in your diet can contribute to heart problems and weight gain. So it's vital to know which fat works for you and which works against.

Monosaturated fat
These provide the good cholesterol (HDL) and help keep down the bad (LDL). They are found in olive oil, groundnut oil, flaxseed oil and avocados and should be used instead of saturated fats at every opportunity. It's particularly good idea to replace butter with olive oil spread.

Saturated fats
These raise cholesterol levels across the board, and as they contain more LDL than HDL present, will do you far more harm than good. Dairy and animal fats – butter, cheese, lard, suet, chicken fat, bacon etc – are rich in saturates, and should be avoided or substituted with monosaturates wherever possible.

Polyunsaturated fats
Opposite to saturated fats, these lower both forms of cholesterol and so are to be encouraged. The essential fatty acids omega-3 and omega-6 are polyunsaturated fats and can be found in, respectively, fish oils, oily fish and olive oil, as well as soya beans, soya spread, sunflower seeds, sunflower oil and corn oil.

Cholesterol in foods
Eggs and shellfish both contain cholesterol, but in such small amounts that, unless that is all you live on, they won't do you any harm.

Trans fats
Nothing boosts your LDL higher than trans fats, which are common in processed foods. There is no safe level for them, so avoid anything that includes 'partially hydrogenized oils' in its list of ingredients.

WHAT IS CHOLESTEROL?

In spite of the bad press it gets, some cholesterol in your body is vital. Cholesterol is a lipid produced by the liver and it's one of the fats that must be present for a number of reasons. Cholesterol is an important factor in the make-up of the body's cells; it is part of the formation of hormones; it carries other fats (triglycerides) through the bloodstream to the tissues and for the formation and maintenance of cell walls; and it facilitates the transportation of fat-soluble vitamins A, D, E and K. Foods that are rich in saturated fats – fatty meat, full-fat dairy, chicken with its skin on – provide a great deal of our cholesterol intake, while, conversely, cholesterol-rich food such as eggs and shellfish won't actually significantly raise the blood's cholesterol levels.

However, while some cholesterol is crucial, it's also a potential killer, as when lipids and triglycerides combine, they form lipoproteins, which fall into two different categories: High Density Lipoprotein (HDL) and Low Density Lipoprotein (LDL). These two compounds have a very different effect within the body: HDL is cholesterol being taken back to the liver for reprocessing after what was needed has been used, while LDL is excess and circulates cholesterol around the arteries. In doing so, it has the potential to leave fat on the artery walls which can harden into life-threatening deposits which restrict the blood flow and can break off to form blood clots.

Because it is impossible to control whether you produce HDL (good cholesterol) or LDL (harmful cholesterol), and the latter will actually make up the vast majority of a person's lipoprotein, it is vital not to take on too much cholesterol in the diet. Only by reducing the total amount can you reduce the volume of potentially harmful LDL. Therefore, it is very important to monitor the amount of cholesterol you are taking on board.

As a diabetic it is essential your diet reflects a low-cholesterol approach. Equally important, is an annual Lipid Panel Screening to check your blood cholesterol level, your levels of HDL, LDL and triglycerides.

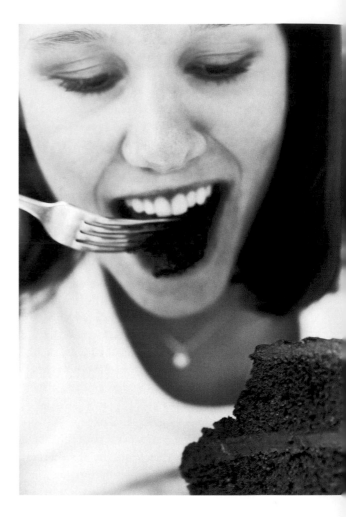

doctor, there will be a degree of leeway within it for you to mix and match starchy and fibrous carbohydrates, provided you maintain a good balance throughout.

One of the best ways to ensure you get the right blend of carbohydrates is to eat plenty of fresh fruit and vegetables. Increasing this intake as a proportion of your diet is vital for weight loss or diabetes control, as it means you will be cutting down on fat and taking on extra vitamins and minerals. Study after study has shown that people with diets highest in fruit and vegetables have the lowest incidences of diabetes, heart complaints and many other illnesses. Maintaining ▶

BUT CAN I DRINK ALCOHOL?

In a word, yes. Provided you're sensible about it, especially if you're an insulin-dependent diabetic. The presence of alcohol on an empty stomach can trigger a hypo as it seriously impairs the liver's ability to cope with low blood glucose. But follow these guidelines, avoid excessive or binge drinking and it will be perfectly safe for you to raise a social glass or two.

■ Don't go over the safe limit of 21-28 units per week for men and 14-21 per week for women – and don't try to store up unit credit thinking you can drink two weeks' worth in one evening.

■ Make at least every other day a 'dry' day.

■ Pace yourself out during the course of the evening and have something to eat with every drink.

■ Beware of low-alcohol drinks, which are often higher in sugar as it hasn't been turned into alcohol.

■ Be aware that diabetic or low-sugar drinks are likely to be higher in alcohol for exactly the opposite reason, so it's probably best to stick to ordinary drinks.

■ Avoid drinking cocktails that contain a lot of sugary ingredients like margarita or pina colada.

■ Always ask for low-calorie mixers.

■ Cutting down on drinking is a sure-fire way to lose weight as the calorific content of alcohol is very high. To avoid a drinker's belly, stick to wine rather than beer or spirits.

■ Red wine is actually a good source of chromium, a mineral vital for controlling diabetes.

a balance is really at the core of all healthy eating plans. For a diabetic to avoid blood sugar spikes, this will mean making sure there is a balance of carbohydrate, protein and fat within each meal and throughout the day. The exact balance will differ depending on a person's size and lifestyle.

Always go for the whole food and fresh food option, avoid as much processed food as you can, and go organic whenever practical. A degree of common sense must be employed when considering sugar or alcohol, and the timing of meals will have to be rebalanced. Insulin-dependent diabetics should time their meals according to when they have their shots, to give the drug time to be absorbed, while some diabetics should eat less more often.

The most important thing to remember, however, is that as a diabetic you can still enjoy your food and stay healthy. whether you're dining out or at home. ▶

PROTEIN POWER

Although the average modern UK diet involves too much protein, it is crucial for body cell renewal and maintenance. It's available to us as vegetable and animal protein, the former being present in nuts, beans and pulses – which is why vegetarians should eat large amounts of these foods – while the latter is found in meat, dairy and fish. Of the two, vegetable protein is recommended to those on a diabetic or weight-loss eating plan, as, unless the meat is very lean and the cheese and milk low-fat, it's likely to contain an unhealthy degree of saturated fat.

It is important that, should you give up meat or dairy, you keep your protein intake up. Make sure your eating plans includes dishes like West Indian-style rice and peas (red beans), tomato and lentil soup and hummus (made from chickpeas). Even the humble peanut butter sandwich will be packed with protein and fibre!

FABULOUS FIBRE

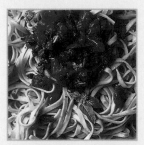

Fibre is the unsung hero of the diabetic's healthy eating plan, As well as playing a big part in glucose release control, it can help to keep weight down. It's no coincidence so many low GI foods, such as pulses and wholemeal flour, are high in fibre.

There are two types of fibre our bodies need: soluble and insoluble. The former, found in fruit and beans, physically swells up in the stomach, which gives you a feeling of being full although you've eaten less. This increase in size also delays the movement of food into the small intestine. Then the soluble fibre breaks down into a thick gel-like substance that slows down carbohydrate and glucose absorption into the intestines . These actions help to prevent any post-meal surges in blood sugar, meaning lower, more regular insulin levels.

Insoluble fibre, found in whole grains, works much more directly, but no less effectively. It takes much longer to chew and that means the brain gets the 'I'm full' message much earlier than it might, as the action of chewing helps trigger the chemical messenger.

Remarkably though, hardly anybody in the UK eats enough fibre. The government recommended minimum is 18 g (0.6 oz), although 24 g (0.8 oz) is the ideal, yet the average Brit consumes a mere12 g (0.4 oz) of this wonder food a day. Simple tips for eating more would be: choose chocolate with nuts in it; opt for fruit pie instead of a slice of cake; change to wholemeal pasta; or swap the cornflakes for Shredded Wheat in the morning.

WHAT DO THEY MEAN BY A SERVING?

Dietary advice recommends foods by the number of servings you should eat per day, while the nutritional advice on labels offers amounts of vitamins and minerals per serving. But how much is a serving? The truth is, it's different for just about everything! These are some of the most common examples for a healthy eating plan suitable for everyone.

FRUIT and VEGETABLES
One serving is:
50 g (2 oz) cooked or raw vegetables
40 (1½ oz) raw salad leaves

180 ml (6 fl oz) fruit or vegetable juice
1 medium-sized piece of fruit

WHOLE GRAINS
One serving is:
1 slice wholemeal bread
100 g (3½ oz) brown rice
60 g (2½ oz) wholemeal pasta

HIGH CALCIUM FOODS
One serving is:
240 ml (8 fl oz) low-fat or skimmed milk
225 g (8 oz) low-fat yoghurt
25 g (1 oz) low-fat cheese

240 ml (8 fl oz) calcium-fortified orange juice

BEANS
One serving is:
100 g (3 ½oz) cooked beans, pulses or lentils

NUTS
One serving is:
Two tablespoons chopped nuts

FISH AND MEAT
One serving is:
75 g (3 oz) cooked fish; 110 g (4 oz) cooked meat or poultry

TOP 10 DIABETES BUSTIN' SUPER FOODS

THE FOODS YOU CAN'T AFFORD TO IGNORE IF YOU WANT TO MAXIMIZE YOUR DIABETES CONTROLLING EATING PLAN.

Garlic
Strengthens the immune system by acting as a natural antibiotic, and is also a powerful anti-fungal agent. For diabetics it has a few added advantages: it lowers all cholesterol in the blood; keeps blood flowing more easily; and has been shown to make a huge difference in the management of blood sugar levels.

Dandelions
Eaten as salad leaves or taken as a supplement, dandelions stimulate the liver for more efficient storing and release of glucose. They also lower blood cholesterol, reduce blood pressure and are a very rich source of fibre.

Peanuts
A very good source of vegetable protein, providing your minimum requirements without the additional risk of saturated fat found in meat and cheese.

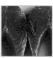

Red chilli peppers
They supercharge the circulatory system by reducing cholesterol levels, thinning the blood and thus protecting against clots. But the big bonus of chilli peppers is that they release the endorphins that trigger pleasure sensors in the brain.

Salmon
The king of the oily fish is a rich source of the essential fatty acid omega-3. This is vital for raising the level of HDL (good cholesterol) and thinning the blood to increase circulation and reduce the risk of clotting.

Freshly ground black pepper
A potent blood purifier and digestive aid, as well as making food taste better it is much harder worker than other peppers.

Olive oil
This should be the only oil you use, as it is so rich in monosaturated fats it can assist in lowering harmful cholesterol levels. Even so, don't use more than you need to.

Bilberries
Bilberries are great for your blood flow. They boost circulation, are anti-clotting and reduce blood vessel wall deposits. The same antioxidant agents they contain in abundance are also particularly effective in maintaining the capillaries around the eyes, and so combat the degenerative eye disorders often associated with diabetes.

Red wine
While being careful not to recommend any form of over-indulgence, red wine is rich in chromium, a mineral that promotes the production of insulin in the pancreas, then assists its absorption into the bloodstream. Chromium is also important in regulating glucose and cholesterol levels.

Root ginger
For centuries, root ginger has been an acknowledged digestive aid and stomach settler. For diabetics, however, it can also help enormously by cutting down blood stickiness, thus reducing any cardio-vascular strain.

WHAT EXACTLY DOES IT SAY ON THE TIN?

DON'T BELIEVE THE HYPE WHEN IT COMES TO YOUR SHOPPING BASKET. FOOD LABELLING CAN BE A MINEFIELD OF MISUNDERSTANDING AND DOWNRIGHT MISINFORMATION, SO IT PAYS TO UNDERSTAND THE JARGON AND SMALL PRINT.

THE WAY FOODS ARE LABELLED IS strictly governed by British and European law, so if you know how the system works, you can be absolutely clear what is in the food you're eating. But when the manufacturers are trying to do everything they can – without flouting the regulations – to persuade you to buy their product, it can be a little confusing. Words like 'pure' make a particular product seem more appealing, but in order to put these words on the packet, the manufacturer has to comply with certain rules. This is what the law says:

■ Everything that goes into a food product must be listed in descending order of weight on the packaging.

■ The label must not be misleading when it describes food as being 'fresh' or 'natural', and must state the correct country of origin, if it is relevant, eg Mexican honey has to originate from Mexico.

■ Labels must be specific about any processes that the food has undergone, be it UHT-treated or irradiated. If a product is fruit-flavoured using artificial flavouring – a yoghurt or jelly, for example – then it can't have a picture of fresh fruit on the box.

■ All manufacturers must include their name and address on the packaging so you can contact them for more information and details about how to store, prepare and cook the product.

If you have any doubts about an item, contact the manufacturer and ask them directly, check with a dietician, or contact the Food Standards Agency (FSA) (see page 156). This is the Government's independent food safety watchdog that protects public health and consumer interests in relation to food. ◻

BIO
Bio is Greek for 'life'. In food terms, it's most often found in yoghurts that claim to have live bacteria or cultures in them. There is no Food Standard Agency rule about what the word 'bio' means or how it should be used on labels.

FREE FROM
By law, alcohol-free beer must contain no more than 0.05 per cent alcohol, but there are no equivalent guidelines for 'gluten-free', 'dairy-free' etc, so it's best to check the ingredients as well as the wording on the front of the packet.

LIGHT OR LITE
There aren't any rules governing how much or how little fat there has to be in a product for it to qualify as being 'light'. A bag of crisps described as light may even have as many calories as the original version, so check the nutritional panel on the packet.

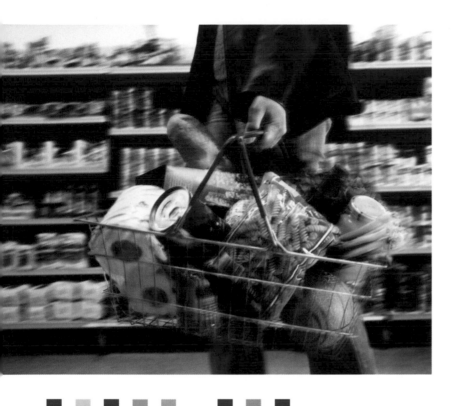

DIABETES-FRIENDLY FOOD

Supermarkets and even chemists stock foods labelled 'suitable for diabetics' or simply 'diabetic'. But Diabetes UK and the Food Standards Agency agree that these products are over-priced and unnecessary. Sticking to a healthy, well-balanced diet that includes plenty of fresh fruit and vegetables, starchy carbohydrates, and only a small amount of sugar, is sound advice for diabetics and non-diabetics alike. As most of the foods labelled 'suitable for diabetics' are sweets and biscuits, you are better off avoiding them anyway, and choosing less processed foods that you can share with your family.

HEALTHY EATING LOGOS
Almost all supermarkets have their own range that they promote as a healthy alternative to the standard products, with fewer calories, less fat or less salt. It's up to each company how they decide what goes into the range, so check with them what the criteria are for a product to be labelled as a 'healthy option' and, as always, read the label.

HEALTH CLAIMS
No foods can be described as treating or curing a health problem — if they did they'd be classified as medicines and be governed by a different set of regulations. They can say that they help or aid your health, for example 'helps maintain a healthy heart', if it is not misleading to do so.

REDUCED LACTOSE/FAT/SALT
The FSA recommend that the term 'reduced' should only be used on products that contain 75 per cent or less of the particular ingredient than the standard version.

NO ADDED SUGAR
Just because a product doesn't have sugar added to it, doesn't mean it doesn't contain sugar. The same goes for foods that are 'unsweetened'. Fruit has a naturally high sugar content, and lactose, which is found in milk, is another source of sugar in food.

LOW-FAT
Manufacturers are not allowed to label their products in a way that could mislead the consumer, but there are no hard and fast rules about what makes something 'low-fat'. The FSA recommends that 'low-fat' foods should contain less than 3 per cent fat, and 'fat-free' should be less than 1.5 per cent. Remember, if something is 85 per cent fat free it actually contains 15 per cent fat.

YOUR GUIDE TO
THE GLYCAEMIC INDEX

BY RATING CARBOHYDRATES BY HOW THEY'LL AFFECT YOUR BLOOD SUGAR,
THE GLYCAEMIC INDEX IS AN INVALUABLE TOOL FOR YOUR EATING PLAN.

THE GLYCAEMIC INDEX HAS BEEN PART of diabetes research for more than 20 years now, and, as recommended by the World Health Organization, has become the accepted basis for dietary blood sugar management. Glycaemic Index (GI) numbers are assigned to carbohydrate-heavy foods – bread, potatoes, fruit, chocolate etc – and ranked by the effect they have on your blood sugar during the two- to three-hour period after eating. The ratings indicate the speed at which the foods are broken down during the digestion process, and how quickly they introduce glucose into the bloodstream.

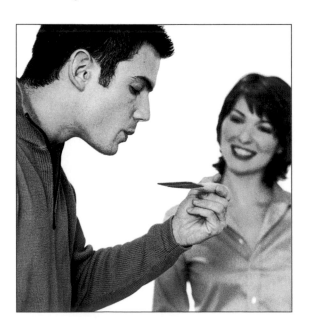

All carbohydrate is eventually metabolized into glucose which will end up in your bloodstream and be absorbed through the muscle cell walls as fuel. However, different foods are broken down at different speeds, meaning that, as glucose release is a gradual process taking place over the entire course of digestion, glucose hits the bloodstream at very different rates. To most people this can prove uncomfortable, but to a diabetic it is potentially hazardous. The speeds can vary from the slow and steady release that is needed for good blood sugar levels management, through to a dumping of glucose so fast it can cause dangerous surges in blood sugar.

The Index identifies which food performs at what rate: the lower the GI number, the lower the risk of that food spiking your blood sugar levels, and the higher the number, the greater the danger. A good rule to follow is a GI number of 55 or less is easy on the system; GI of 56-70 will only marginally raise the level; while anything over 70 can send blood sugar levels soaring with dizzying speed.

While every GI number is relevant to your healthy eating plan, don't think you need to completely cut out all high-GI foods. Using our handy guide to a wide selection of popular foods, you can organize balanced eating plans that won't veer too far in one direction. Also, don't assume what might appear to be obvious with certain foods, or base your dietary choices on GI alone.

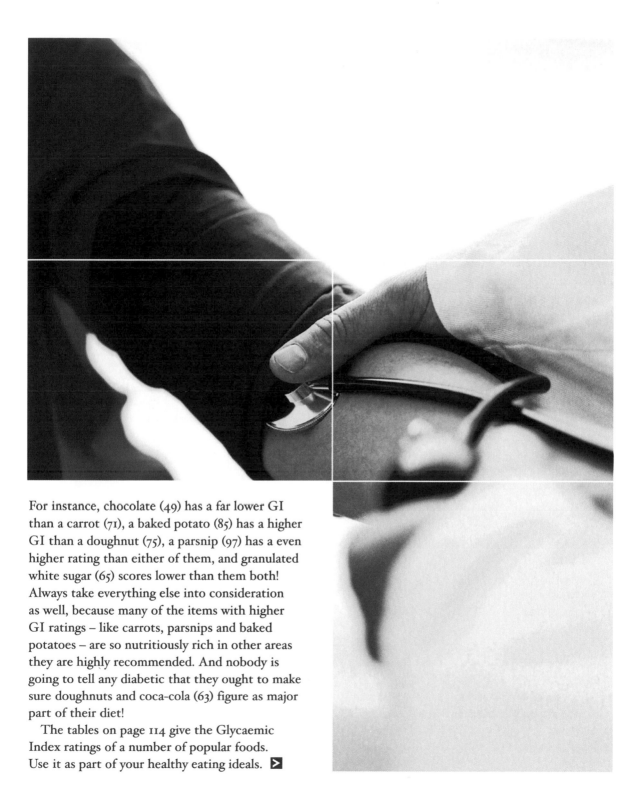

For instance, chocolate (49) has a far lower GI than a carrot (71), a baked potato (85) has a higher GI than a doughnut (75), a parsnip (97) has a even higher rating than either of them, and granulated white sugar (65) scores lower than them both! Always take everything else into consideration as well, because many of the items with higher GI ratings – like carrots, parsnips and baked potatoes – are so nutritiously rich in other areas they are highly recommended. And nobody is going to tell any diabetic that they ought to make sure doughnuts and coca-cola (63) figure as major part of their diet!

The tables on page 114 give the Glycaemic Index ratings of a number of popular foods. Use it as part of your healthy eating ideals. ▶

GLYCAEMIC INDEX

**GLYCAEMIC INDEX
OF LESS THAN 55**
Glucose will be released
slowly into the bloodstream

Low-fat yoghurt	
(artificially sweetened)	14
Peanuts	14
Plums	24
Grapefruit	25
Dried apricots	31
Soya milk	31
Skimmed milk	32
Apples	36
Pears	36
Wholemeal spaghetti	37
Tomato soup	38
Apple juice	41
Spaghetti (refined flour)	41
All Bran	42
Grapes	43
Oranges	43
Pineapple juice	46
Long grain rice	47
Grapefruit juice	48
Tinned baked beans	48
Chocolate	49
Kiwi fruit	52
Banana	53
Stoneground	
wholemeal bread	53
Crisps	54

**GLYCAEMIC INDEX
OF BETWEEN 56 AND 70**
Glucose will be released quickly
but still safely into the bloodstream

Brown rice	55
Oatmeal cookies	55
Popcorn	55
Sweetcorn	55
White rice	56
Pitta bread	57
Blueberry muffin	59
Bran muffin	60
Cheese pizza	60
Ice cream	61
Coca-cola	63
Macaroni cheese	64
Granulated white	
sugar	65
Cous cous	65
Instant oatmeal	66
Pineapple	66
Taco shells	68
Wholemeal bread	69
White bread	70

GLYCAEMIC INDEX OF OVER 70
Glucose will be released very
quickly into the bloodstream

Carrots	71
Bagels	72
Watermelon	72
Honey	73
Mashed potatoes	73
Bran Flakes	74
Doughnuts	75
Chips	76
Rice cakes	82
Rice Krispies	82
Cornflakes	84
Baked potato	85
French bread	95
Parsnips	97
Dried dates	103

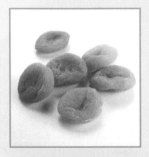
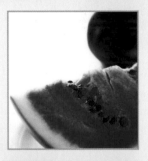
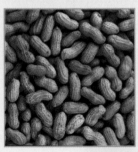
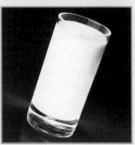

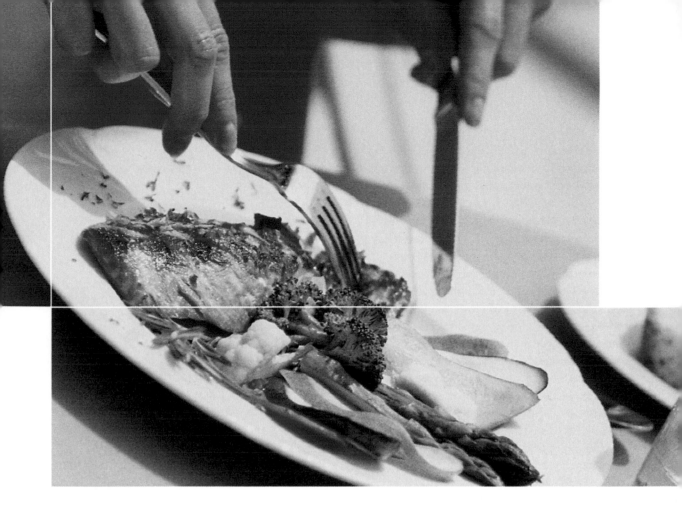

DINING OUT

THERE'S NO REASON WHY ANY RESTAURANT SHOULD BE OFF LIMITS IF YOU'VE BEEN DIAGNOSED WITH DIABETES. ALL THAT'S REQUIRED IS A BIT OF EXTRA THOUGHT.

EATING OUT AS A DIABETIC IS SIMPLY a matter of being sensible rather than total abstinence. For many people, going for a meal at a restaurant, grabbing a takeaway on the way home from work or taking the kids for a fast-food treat is an integral part of today's lifestyle, and people with diabetes are no different. Food prepared outside the home shouldn't be thought of as out of bounds for a diabetic. Instead, here's how you can make the most of restaurant dining and takeaway menus without too much inconvenience or compromise.

Choosing a meal out isn't very different from planning a meal at home, as most reputable restaurants will use fresh ingredients, meaning there won't be too many hidden dangers. The logical way to make your choice would be to ask yourself 'Is that something I would cook and eat at home?' However, it's often the choices on offer that present the biggest hurdles to a diabetic diner as they clearly aren't what you would cook and eat at home – which is why you've gone out to eat in the first place! So you need to think carefully about your selection. ▶

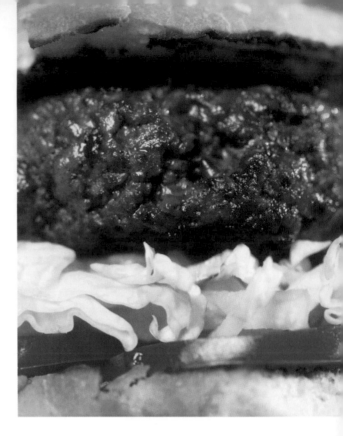

If you intend to go out for a special lavish meal or to eat at a friend's house, remember to keep a balance between that meal and what you eat on either side of it. If you're likely to increase sugar and fat intake at that meal, cut it down elsewhere, and approach your calorie counting as a total for the day rather than meal by meal. Try not to go out to dinner too hungry, as the temptation to fill up on rolls and butter may prove too much. And make sure you tell anybody who invites you to their home for dinner about your condition – there's no need to feel any more embarrassed than you would if you were a vegetarian or had a nut allergy. You're out to enjoy yourself, so don't fret too much about what you're about to eat because increasing your stress levels will definitely not help your digestion or your blood pressure.

Upmarket dining

The trick is to avoid heavy sauces and meals that contain a lot of fat. Although top class restaurants seem to offer a greater proportion of rich food, the fact that it is cooked to order makes it easier to have things prepared in a certain way, without any less-healthy aspects of the dish that might appear on the menu. Which illustrates how important it is to talk to the restaurant staff and ask what a meal contains, how it is cooked and if it is possible to have it made in a slightly different way. Also, let them know your condition as their kitchen might have experience in catering for customers with diabetes, and if it is an establishment you go to frequently they might start thinking of how best to cater to your needs. Restaurant staff should be knowledgeable about what is in the dishes on the menu, and willing to accommodate your requirements – if that's not the case or they are unwilling to discuss it with you, then leave and give that place a wide berth in the future.

As regards the sweet trolley, you can enjoy the occasional sinful dessert, providing you don't go for double helpings! A small amount of extra sugar should be all right because, if it goes down on top of the rest of the meal and mixes with the food in your stomach, it will be absorbed quite slowly into your system.

Hamburger heaven

The golden rule of burger bar dining is to avoid the super-size option! Portions in major hamburger chains have been getting bigger and bigger, so when the young charmer behind the counter smiles and asks you if you want that 'super-sized', remember that increasing your portions now may be directly related to shortening your lifespan – and say no.

If you keep to this rule then intermittent hamburger meals shouldn't do you any harm, especially if you follow these simple guidelines:
- Cheese and/or bacon on your burger will almost double the calories – so don't have it.
- Ask for your burger without the sauce.
- Don't assume the veggie burger is healthier – it will still have been fried.
- Try to avoid too many extras: onion rings and

fries will send the fat levels soaring, and the fruit pies are essentially sugar bombs.

■ Order diet drinks as they will have much less sugar than regular – 330 ml (11.6 fl oz) of most colas contains around 35 g (1.2 oz) of sugar.

■ If there's a choice, opt for fat chips rather than skinny-cut fries; the total surface area of a portion of the former will be smaller and therefore will have absorbed less fat.

■ Drink water with your meal, as it will curb your appetite and your thirst for those extra calories.

Fish and chips

Whatever goodness you could get from the fish will be pretty much cancelled out by how it's cooked and served. To limit the amount of fat you consume, try not to eat the batter, or at least only eat one side of it. With fat chip-shop chips, the kindest thing you can say is that they are doing you less harm than the skinny fries you might get in a burger chain! Simply ask for less – chip shop portions are far bigger than they need to be, so either share one bag between two of you or stop them serving you so many.

Kebab

If you fancy a kebab, a shish, particularly a chicken shish, will be better for you than a donner (you might think it's made from lean lamb, but look at the fat oozing out of the meat as it cooks). Ask for a generous helping of salad too.

Indian and Chinese

In both cases, opt for steamed or boiled dishes rather than fried ones, and opt for vegetable, chicken or prawn instead of pork, beef or lamb. As regards the rice, pilau rice is fried, and, like Chinese special fried rice, it has many more calories than boiled rice. Likewise the soft noodles are boiled or steamed – the crispy noodles will have been deep fried. In an Indian restaurant be wary of the desserts and sweets as they are notoriously sugary. Be careful of set menus too; they often give you more food than you want, and limit your choice.

Pizza precautions

Unfortunately, like hamburgers, pizzas are not recommended as everyday food for a diabetic. So while you can enjoy one occasionally, you need to be careful. Stay away from thick crust pizzas as their calorie rating will be way up the dial and opt for vegetable toppings rather than ham or pepperoni. Also, avoid the temptation of extra cheese, and ask if they do a healthy eating

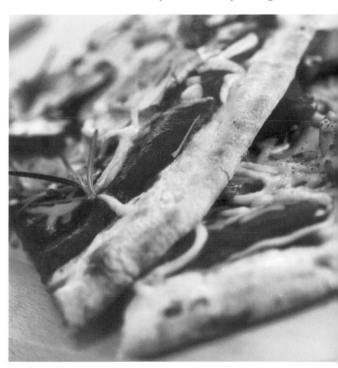

pizza using reduced-fat cheese and a choice of vegetable, fish or seafood toppings.

If the pizza restaurant also serves pasta, then opt for that. Even pasta made with processed white flour will be easier on your system than most pizzas, as its GI rating of 41 compares favourably with the most basic pizza's 60 (see the Glycaemic Index, page 114). ◘

THE ONLY SHOPPING LIST YOU'LL NEED

We've talked a great deal about different sorts of fat, the Glycaemic Index, complex and simple carbs, cholesterol and so on, but where all this really counts is in your fridge and kitchen cupboards. Follow this handy list when you're doing your food shopping and you'll be able to eat healthily and safely, and stay in control of your diabetes. Of course, don't forget to put the occasional treat on your list, as by following the guidelines elsewhere in this chapter there's no reason why you can't let yourself go from time to time. You deserve it!

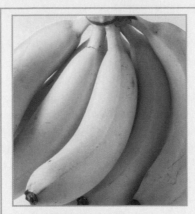

IN A COOL DRY PLACE

Bananas

Grapefruit

Oranges

Raisins

Nuts (almonds, peanuts, walnuts, pine nuts, pecans, pistachios)

Seeds (sunflower, sesame)

Melon (honeydew, cantaloupe, watermelon)

Plums

Sweet potatoes

Butternut squash

Garlic

Onions

Cabbage (red or green)

Carrots

Cauliflower

Raisins

Coconuts

IN THE FRIDGE

Olive oil spread

Reduced-fat cheese

Eggs

Fruit juice (orange, apple, grapefruit, pineapple)

Skimmed milk

Yoghurt (natural, low-fat)

Sour cream (reduced-fat)

Mayonnaise (reduced-fat)

Olives in brine

Strawberries

Grapes

Apples

Lemons

Kiwi fruit

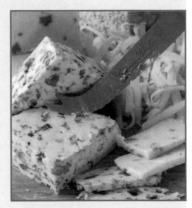

Fresh broccoli

Fresh spinach

Greens

Brussel sprouts

Mangetout

Red, green or yellow peppers

Mushrooms

Courgettes

Aubergines

Fresh herbs (parsley, basil, thyme, sage, mint, tarragon, oregano)

IN THE FREEZER

Sweetcorn

Broccoli

THE ONLY SHOPPING LIST YOU'LL NEED

Green beans
Peas
Salmon
Kippers
Whole trout
Prawns
Bacon
Veggie burgers

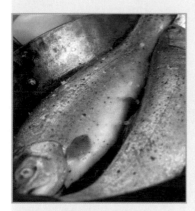

Lean beef (sirloin and fillet
  steak, mince, roasting joints)
Pork chops
Lamb cutlets
Chicken pieces (skinless
  breast or thighs)
Whole chicken
Turkey (breast or cutlets)
Wholemeal bread
Wholemeal tortillas
Wholemeal muffins

IN THE CUPBOARD
Dried apricots
Dried mushrooms
Dried herbs (parsley,
  basil, thyme, sage, mint,
  tarragon, oregano)

Tinned fish (salmon, sardines,
  pilchards in oil, anchovies,
  tuna in brine)
Tinned soup (lentil, chicken,
  vegetable or tomato)
Tinned tomatoes
Passata or thick tomato juice
Tomato sauce (with no
  added sugar)
Dried beans/pulses (red kidney
  beans, black eye peas, lentils,
  haricots, chickpeas)
Baked beans (with no added
  sugar)
Wholemeal flour
Wholemeal bread flour
Wholemeal pasta (various
  shapes)
Dried noodles
Brown rice
Cous cous

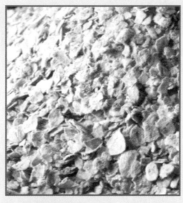

Pudding rice
Wholegrain crackers
Porridge oats
Hot-pepper sauce
Pesto

Soy sauce
Worcestershire sauce
Wholegrain mustard
Whole black peppercorns
Sea salt
Dried spices (ground ginger,
  cinnamon, nutmeg)
Vinegar (balsamic, cider,
  red wine, white wine)
Brown sugar
Peanut butter (crunchy
  or smooth)
Olive oil
Sesame oil
Tea (green, black and fruit)
Herbal infusions
Unsweetened cocoa powder

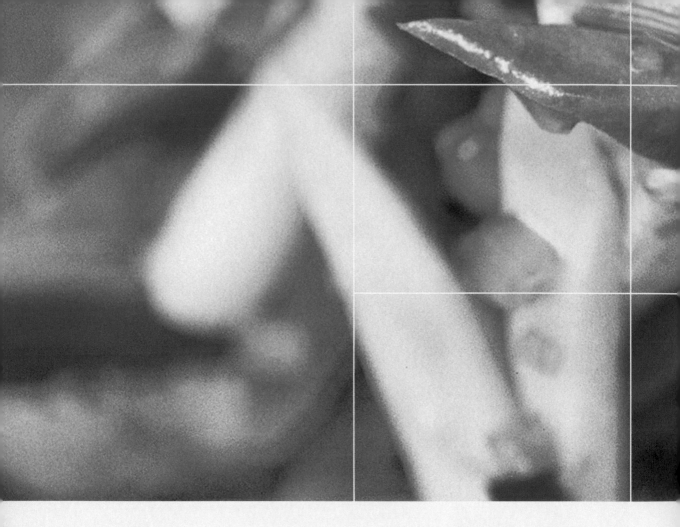

THE OUTSMART
DIABETES
COOKBOOK

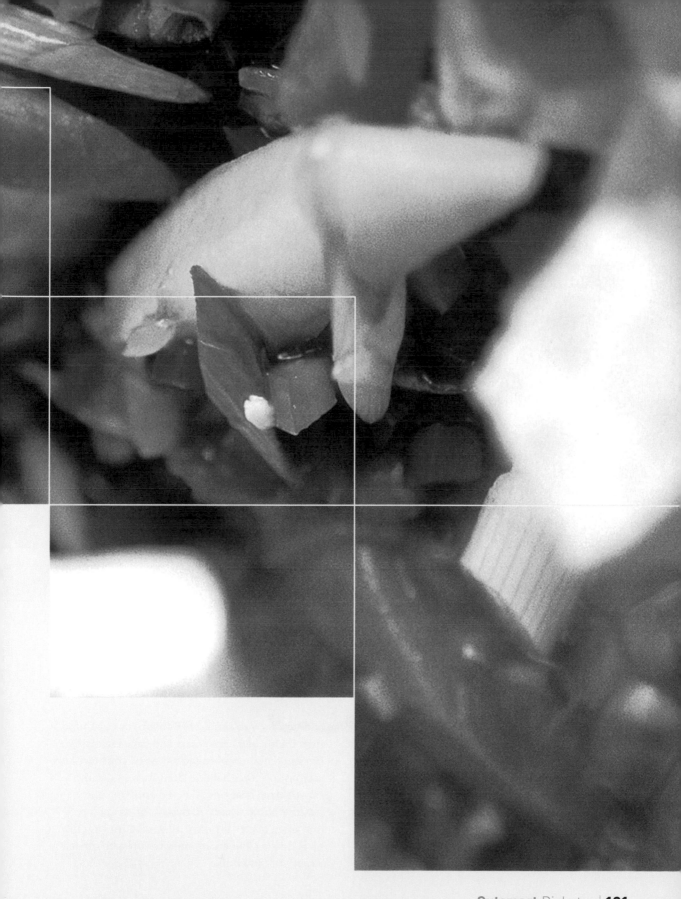

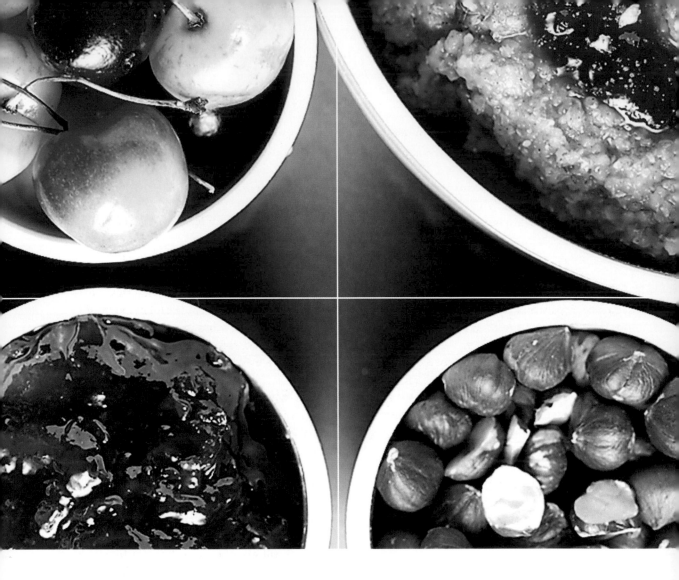

BEFORE YOU START

WITH THESE DELICIOUS AND CONVENIENT RECIPE IDEAS, FIGHTING DIABETES, AND STAYING HEALTHY IN GENERAL, HAS NEVER BEEN SO ENJOYABLE.

THE RECIPES ON THE FOLLOWING PAGES are simply a starting-point for how to adjust your eating habits to menus that are as good to eat as they are good for you.

The most important thing to remember is that as long as you follow the guidelines discussed in *The Food Factor* chapter (see page 100) you can be as adventurous as you like. Provided you remain within the essential balances of dry goods

and liquids, you should feel free to swap around ingredients and create new and exciting tastes. Or you could simply adapt some of your favourite recipes to more diabetic-friendly versions by substituting traditional ingredients for more health-conscious alternatives – for example, exchange butter for olive oil spread for example, or instead of full cream milk try using a low-fat variety or soya milk.

It is important to remember that not all the ingredients behave in exactly the same way and, as quantities may need to be adjusted accordingly, an amount of trial and error may be involved. But don't let that put you off. The important thing is you get into the kitchen and prepare your own food from fresh, health-promoting ingredients as one more way of taking control of your diabetes.

EQUIPMENT

These recipes use everyday equipment that can be found in most people's kitchens. However, if you are contemplating doing a lot of cooking, it's worth investing in a heavy duty food processor and a good set of scales. As regards smaller items, a garlic press is a good idea, as is a lemon squeezer or citrus press – because juicing lemons or oranges in a juicer or processor pulverizes the skin in between the segments, it can give the juice a bitter taste. Finally, a zester will be worth its weight in gold when it comes to recipes that call for the zest (the coloured part of the peel) of any citrus fruit.

SUGAR

Several of the following recipes contain small amounts of sugar and, unless totally impractical, we use unrefined brown sugar. Sugar can be part of a diabetic's healthy eating plan provided it is managed correctly and taken instead of and not as well as other carbohydrate foods (see page 103). That said, wherever possible we've used fruit as a natural sweetener and avoided adding sugar, honey or molasses.

WHOLEMEAL FLOUR

All the flour we use is wholemeal, which has a coarser texture and a more distinct flavour. The most important reason, however, is that it also contains more nutritional and fibre value than white flour, which has been refined.

Be warned though, wholemeal flour, especially the organic variety, is notoriously temperamental and the same recipe may turn out slightly differently each time you use it. You have to be sensitive to its performance as you use it and adjust liquid quantities accordingly.

SEA SALT AND FRESHLY GROUND BLACK PEPPER

In all our recipes that call for pepper as seasoning, we insist on freshly ground black pepper. This is because when used fresh from the peppercorn, it is a powerful blood purifier – plus, of course, it has its own distinctive flavour, We use sea salt from a grinder because not only is it unprocessed but it tastes much saltier.

JUICES AND ZEST

All citrus juices used in the recipes should be freshly squeezed, as it is the only way to ensure maximum nutritional benefit and the best taste.

PASTA

In each of our pasta recipes we recommend wholemeal pasta – pasta made with wholemeal flour. Although it's not compulsory, and these recipes will work just as well with white flour pasta, the wholemeal variety is much better for diabetics because the high fibre content slows down digestion, meaning it has a far lower Glycaemic Index (see page 112) than pasta made with refined flour.

And while it may be a bit chewier than regular pasta, not only does this repay with a far higher flavour, but the increased chewing will serve to reduce your appetite, meaning you eat less of it without feeling hungry.

ORGANIC

We recommend using organic produce at every available opportunity as the taste will always be so much more exciting. In addition, it will be free from chemicals and is far more likely to retain the nutrients and vitamins that it is supposed to contain.

SOUPS & STARTERS

MOST OF THESE FIRST COURSE IDEAS CAN ALSO BE SERVED UP AS LUNCH DISHES OR LIGHT DINNERS.

ROAST PARSNIP AND CORIANDER SOUP

Use plenty of pepper in this soup and it will be better than central heating on those cold winter evenings.

900 g (2 lb) fresh parsnips
1 large bunch fresh coriander
3 large cloves garlic
1 medium onion
sea salt and freshly ground black pepper

■ Peel and chop parsnips into large pieces. Place on baking tray, drizzle with olive oil, season with salt and pepper and roast in a hot oven until soft, but starting to brown.

■ Sweat (cook gently without colouring and in its own juices) the roughly chopped onion and the crushed cloves of garlic.

■ Place in blender with roughly chopped coriander leaves, barely cover with vegetable stock and blend until smooth.

■ Pour into a large saucepan, rinse out blender with stock into the saucepan, and on a low heat, correct consistency by adding more stock as it is required.

■ Check seasoning and serve garnished with a sprig of coriander or a swirl of low-fat cream.

BROCCOLI SOUP WITH CHEESE

Children love this, and it's a sneaky-but-easy way to get them to eat a big portion of broccoli without actually realizing it.

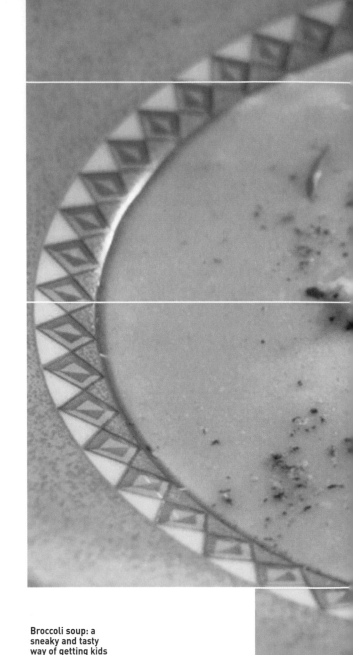

Broccoli soup: a sneaky and tasty way of getting kids to eat nutritious vegetables.

2 large heads of broccoli
115 g (4 oz) low-fat Cheddar cheese
3 large cloves garlic
1 medium onion
sea salt and freshly ground black pepper

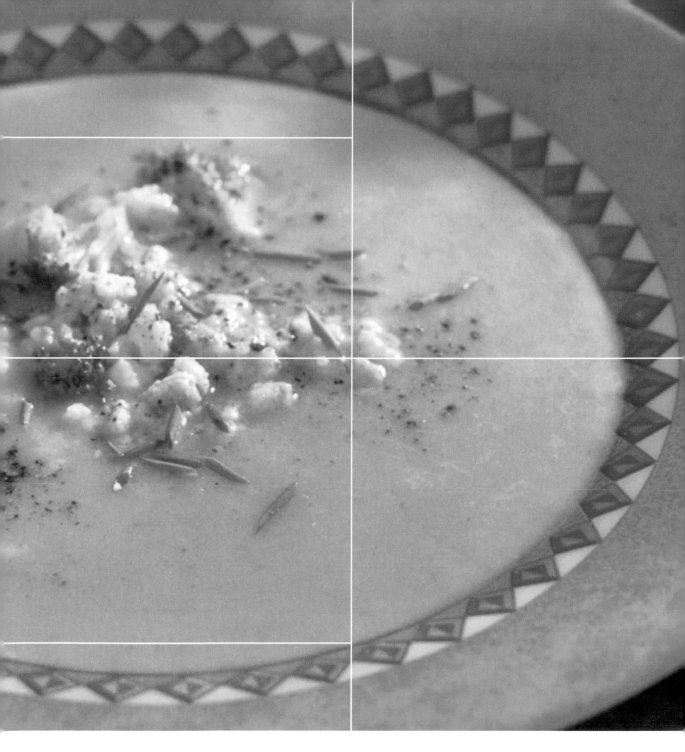

■ Break off broccoli florets and roughly chop stalks. Place in a large lidded saucepan with roughly chopped onion, crushed garlic cloves and salt and pepper.

■ With the lid on, gently cook on a very low heat, until everything is soft (approx 15 minutes). If the broccoli is very fresh, you won't need to start it off with vegetable stock or water in the pan as enough juice should come out of it to stop it burning, but if it is a few days old and therefore a bit drier, add a ladleful of stock or water.

■ When cooked, place the vegetables and the liquid in a blender, barely cover with stock and blend until smooth. ▶

■ Return to the same pan and, on a low heat, adjust the consistency by adding more stock.
■ Check seasoning and serve generously garnished with grated cheese – the soup should be hot enough to start melting the cheese.

GAZPACHO
This is the perfect summer soup – light, crisp and often unexpectedly cold.

1 kg (2.2 lb) very ripe vine tomatoes
½ cucumber
2 red peppers
1 medium onion, roughly chopped
3 cloves garlic
2 tbsp balsamic vinegar

Gazpacho: a refreshing and delicious soup served very cold.

120 ml (¼ pt) olive oil
1 tbsp flat parsley leaves
sea salt and freshly ground black pepper
300 ml (½ pt) vegetable stock
Tabasco sauce
juice of 1 lime
small bunch of chives

■ Peel and remove the seeds from the tomatoes and cucumber and roughly chop. Remove seeds from red peppers and roughly chop.
■ Place in a bowl with crushed garlic cloves, onion, roughly chopped parsley, vinegar, lime juice, olive oil and salt and pepper. Cover and leave to stand at least overnight.
■ Put in blender with stock and purée into a smooth soup.

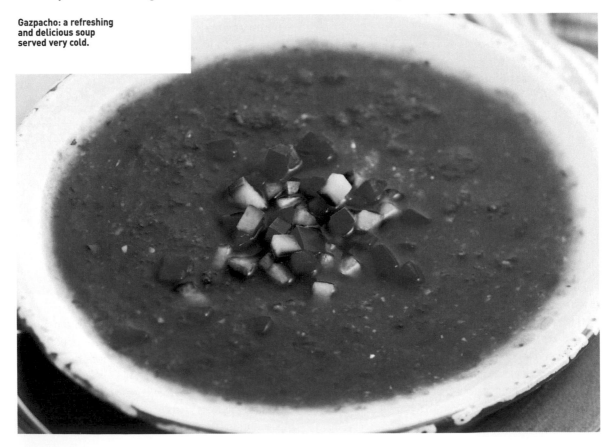

■ Return to a cleaned bowl, season to taste with Tabasco sauce and chill in fridge.
■ Serve in bowls garnished with chopped chives and, if desired, a swirl of low-fat cream.

Gazpacho should be served ice-cold, so bring it to the table with the soup bowls standing in larger dishes covered with crushed ice.

TOMATO & BASIL BRUSCHETTA
This can work as a starter on small pieces of toast, or be served in larger portions as a light meal in its own right.

3 large vine tomatoes
a handful of fresh basil leaves
1 bulb garlic
3 tbsp olive oil
4 slices wholemeal bread, approximately 1.5 cm (½ in) thick
freshly ground black pepper
sea salt
fresh parsley

■ Toast the bread on both sides and put each piece on a separate side plate. Halve or quarter appropriately.
■ Chop the tomato flesh into 1 cm (½ in) cubes (they needn't be peeled) and place it, pips and all, into a large mixing bowl.
■ Roughly cut the basil leaves into approximately the same size and add to tomatoes.
■ Peel the garlic cloves and chop as finely as possible without squashing into a paste. Add to the mix.
■ Sprinkle with the olive oil, season with salt and pepper and mix thoroughly with a metal spoon, being careful not to purée the tomato.
■ Spoon equally on to toast slices, heaping it up and garnishing with parsley. (The parsley will go a long way to reducing garlic breath!)

If this dish is being prepared a long way in advance of serving, mix the tomato, basil, garlic and pepper in a covered bowl, but do not add the salt until just before serving as it will draw the water out of the tomatoes. Then drizzle the oil on the toast rather than add it to the mix.

STUFFED TOMATOES
This can be served either cold, or hot as an attractive vegetable dish.

4 large fresh vine tomatoes
1 green pepper
1 yellow pepper
1 red pepper
60 g (2 oz) fresh French beans
1 small onion
2 cloves garlic
1 tbsp rinsed capers
1 tbsp of basil leaves
1 tbsp flat parsley leaves
2 tbsp olive oil
1 tbsp white wine vinegar
sea salt
freshly ground black pepper

■ Peel tomatoes and cut off tops. Carefully remove seeds by scooping out with a teaspoon.
■ Finely chop onion and garlic, and cook off gently in medium-sized pan in a small amount of olive oil.
■ Remove seeds from the peppers, chop into small squares and add to onions along with the beans (cut into 1 cm/½ in lengths).
■ Remove from heat when starting to soften, but still far from cooked through and set aside to cool.
■ Combine with roughly chopped capers, basil and parsley.
■ Stir in oil and vinegar and season.
■ Generously fill tomatoes with the mixture and replace tops before serving. ◻

PASTA DISHES

MOST OF THESE RECIPES CAN BE MADE WITH ANY SHAPE OF PASTA, SO FEEL FREE TO USE YOUR FAVOURITE TYPES. HOWEVER, ALL DRY PASTA WILL BE SUBJECT TO THE SAME COOKING PROCESS.

Cooking basic pasta
- 75 g (3 oz) dry pasta per portion
- FIll a large saucepan with salted water and bring to the boil.
- Place the pasta into boiling water. If you are using spaghetti, gently ease it down into the water as it softens.
- Stir pasta as water quickly returns to the boil, then turn down to simmer.
- Test individual pieces to see if cooked — they should be soft on the outside but with some resistance (but NOT hard) on the inside. Drain, combine with sauce or garnish and serve.
- If not being served immediately refresh (cool down) under running cold water, drain again and store in fridge until use. Reheat by immersing briefly in boiling water.

Don't hurl pasta against the wall to see if it sticks (if it does, it's cooked) unless you're very sure of what you're doing and have a very tolerant cleaning lady!

FIESTA PASTA SALAD
This tangy pasta dish can pack a kick so be careful with the hot-pepper sauce. It's even more potent if chilled overnight and served cold the next day.

150 g (5 oz) mixed vegetable juice
2 tbsp lime juice
½-1 tsp hot-pepper sauce ▷

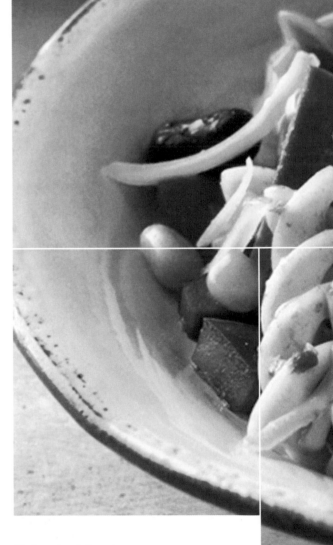

Fiesta pasta salad: a spicy dish that'll put some fire into your dinner party.

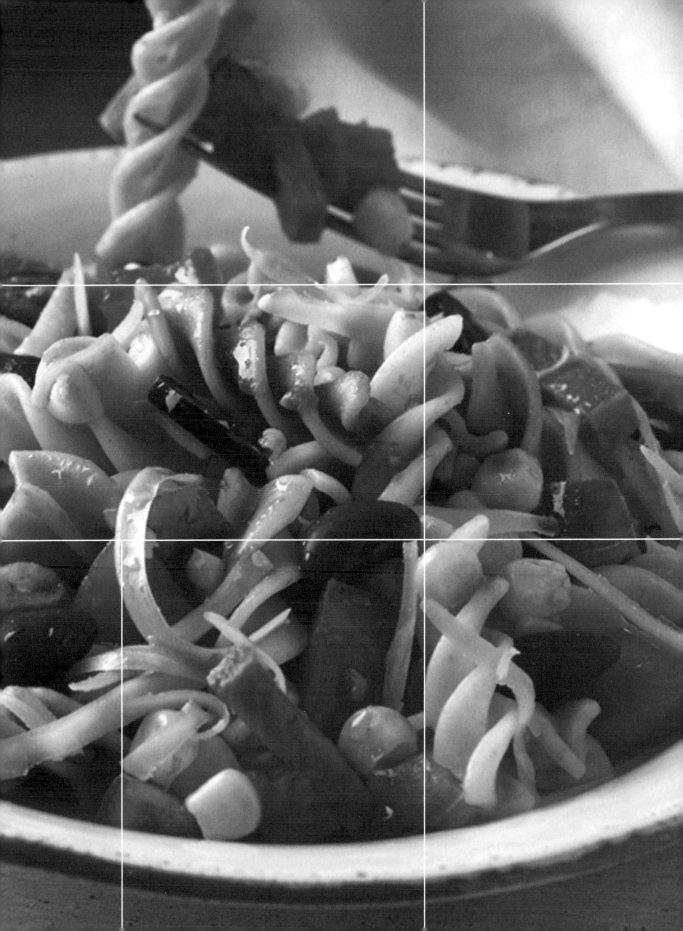

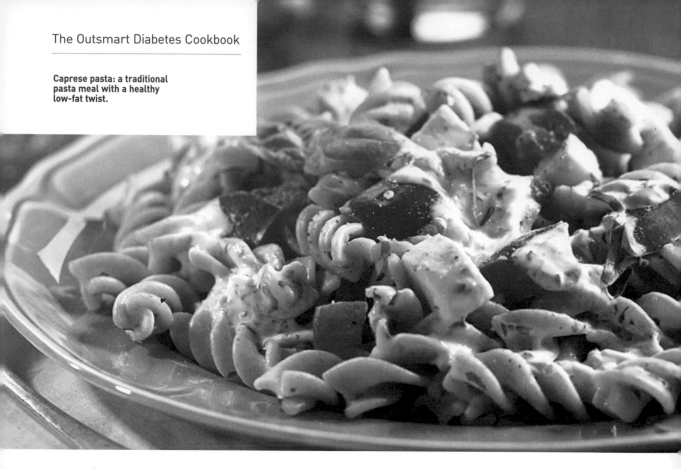

Caprese pasta: a traditional pasta meal with a healthy low-fat twist.

2 large cloves garlic, minced

½ tsp sugar

¼ tsp ground cumin

¼ tsp sea salt

225 g (8 oz) corkscrew pasta, cooked and drained

75 g (3 oz) turkey slices, cut into strips

400 g (14 oz) tinned kidney beans, rinsed and drained

225 g (8 oz) frozen sweetcorn, thawed

110 g (4 oz) grated low-fat Cheddar cheese

3 plum tomatoes, chopped

3 spring onions, sliced

50 g (2 oz) sliced pitted black olives

■ In a large bowl, combine the vegetable juice, lime juice, ½ tsp of hot-pepper sauce, garlic, sugar, cumin and salt. Whisk to mix.
■ Add the pasta, turkey strips, kidney beans, sweetcorn, Cheddar cheese, tomatoes, spring onions and sliced olives.
■ Toss to mix. Taste and add up to ½ tsp more of the hot-pepper sauce, if desired.

CAPRESE PASTA
A traditional pasta dish that enjoys a healthy twist with the inclusion of low-fat yoghurt.

350 g (12 oz) wholemeal fusilli pasta

180 ml (6 fl oz) low-fat natural yoghurt

2 large cloves garlic

1 tbsp olive oil

sea salt and freshly ground black pepper

1 tbsp fresh basil leaves

2 large vine tomatoes

175 g (6 oz) low-fat mozzarella cheese

1 tbsp flat parsley

1 tbsp balsamic vinegar

■ Cook, refresh and drain the pasta (see page 128). While it is cooking, put yoghurt, garlic, oil, salt and pepper and basil leaves in a blender and purée until smooth.
■ Peel and halve tomatoes, and cut flesh into cubes. Cube mozzarella to approximately the same size. Roughly chop parsley.
■ In a small mixing bowl, toss tomatoes, cheese

and parsley in the vinegar.

■ In a large mixing bowl combine pasta and yoghurt dressing.

■ Divide into serving dishes and top with the tomato, cheese and parsley garnish.

This can be served as above – cold as a salad – or as a hot dish, in which case do not refresh the pasta, merely drain it and gently warm both the dressing and garnish in the microwave immediately before use.

FRESH PESTO SAUCE

Although it will always be far more convenient to buy good quality pesto sauce pre-prepared in jars, nothing quite beats the taste of home-made pesto, especially as you will be relatively free to adapt the ingredients to your own preference.

In this recipe, for instance, the addition of chopped pine nuts gives the pesto extra taste.

3 large cloves garlic
2 tbsp olive oil
sea salt and freshly ground black pepper
1 tbsp flat parsley leaves
3 tbsp fresh basil leaves
2 tbsp toasted pine nuts (or walnuts)

■ In blender, purée garlic, olive oil and salt and pepper and empty into mixing bowl.

■ Chop parsley, basil and nuts into small pieces – you should be able to see and taste the herbs and nuts in the sauce, but not have to do too much chewing – and add to purée

■ Mix well and either combine with hot cooked pasta or store in a sealed container in the fridge. Can be kept for a few weeks. ◘

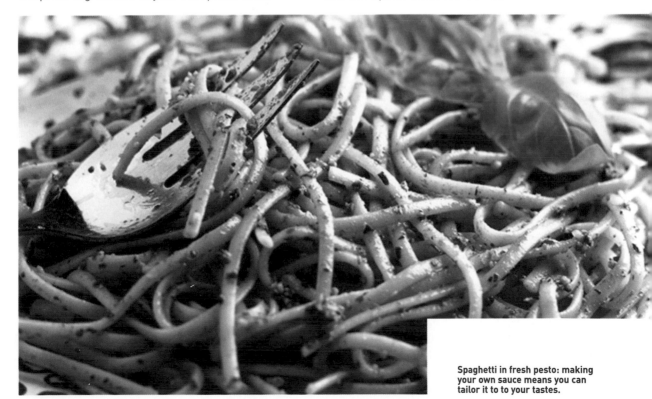

Spaghetti in fresh pesto: making your own sauce means you can tailor it to to your tastes.

MAIN COURSES

NOT ONLY ARE THESE GOOD FOR HEALTHY FAMILY MEALS, BUT WITH EXTRA ATTENTION PAID TO PRESENTATION THEY WON'T BE OUT OF PLACE AT THE SWANKIEST DINNER PARTIES.

GRILLED SWORDFISH WITH BLUEBERRY SALSA

If you can't get swordfish steaks, tuna makes a delicious alternative.

4 x 175 g (6 oz) swordfish steaks
225 g (8 oz) blueberries
225 g (8 oz) watermelon flesh
1 small vine tomato
1 small red onion
1 yellow pepper
1 red pepper
1 jalepeño pepper
2 tbsp fresh basil leaves
2 limes
1 orange
6 spring onions
2 large cloves garlic
1 tbsp olive oil
sea salt and freshly ground black pepper

■ Seed and chop tomato into cubes; likewise the watermelon flesh, yellow pepper, jalepeño pepper, red onion and basil leaves. Seed, halve and roast red pepper, then cut into squares. Combine in bowl with blueberries and refrigerate for at least two hours

■ Grate lime and orange zest into a flat dish. Squeeze in lime and half of orange, add sliced spring onions, finely chopped garlic, olive oil and salt and pepper. Mix well, add fish, coat in the mixture and leave to marinade for at least an hour.

■ Take salsa out of fridge 15 minutes before serving to bring it to room temperature. ▶

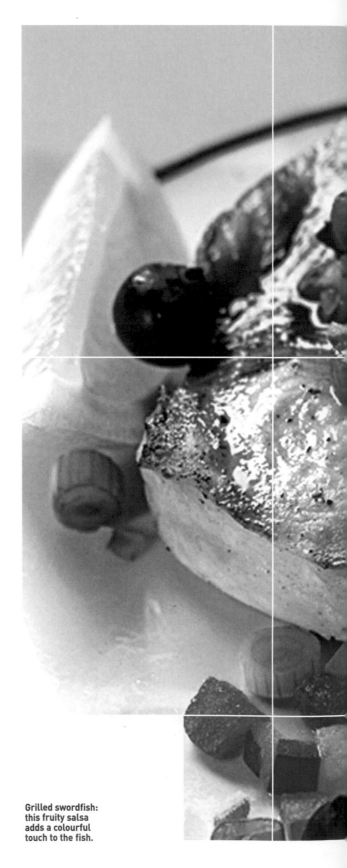

Grilled swordfish: this fruity salsa adds a colourful touch to the fish.

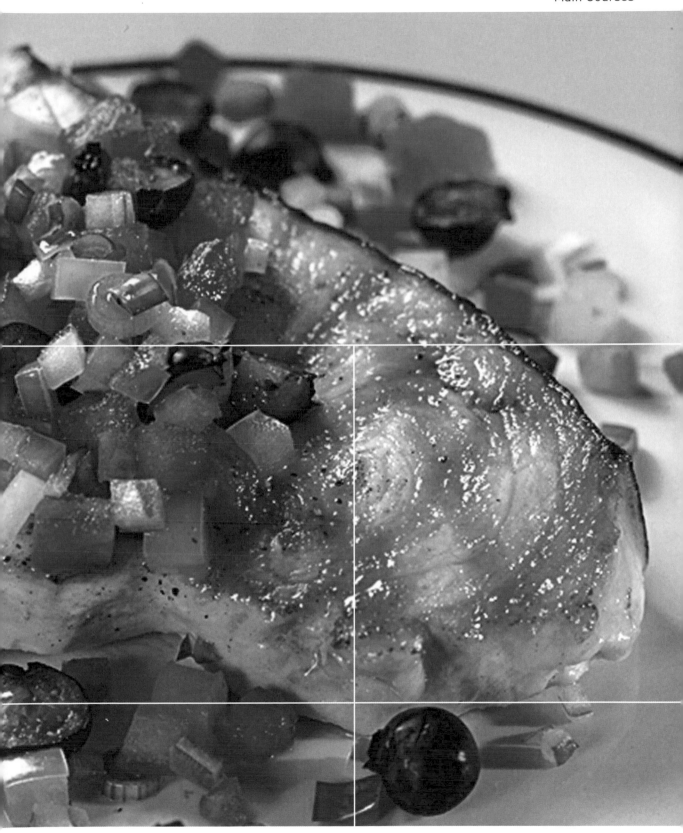

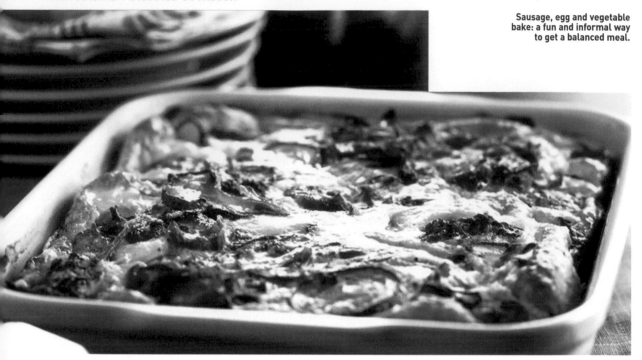

Sausage, egg and vegetable bake: a fun and informal way to get a balanced meal.

■ Remove fish from marinade and place under grill, skin side up, for about four minutes. Turn and return to grill to cook until the fish browns and begins to flake.

■ Serve coated in the blueberry salsa.

SAUSAGE, EGG AND VEGETABLE BAKE

This makes a wonderful, informal family meal.

450 g (1 lb) Italian sausage
1 tbsp olive oil
2 courgettes
1 large aubergine
1 red pepper
1 green pepper
1 red onion
1 large clove garlic
freshly ground sea salt and black pepper
7 eggs
120 ml (4 fl oz) low-fat milk
50 g (2 oz) grated Parmesan cheese

■ Remove any casing from the sausage, cut into 1 cm (½ in) thick slices and fry until half cooked.

■ Drain fat and spread sausage pieces over the bottom of an ovenproof baking dish.

■ Heat olive oil in same pan and quickly fry sliced vegetables and finely chopped garlic until starting to brown but not yet fully cooked.

■ Drain vegetables and pour over sausage slices, season with salt and pepper.

■ In a large mixing bowl, combine eggs, milk and Parmesan cheese, season with salt and pepper and pour over vegetables.

■ Bake in a moderate-to-hot oven for 40—45 mins until eggs are set.

■ Cut into squares to serve.

TROUT WITH ALMONDS AND TARRAGON

The cooking method and the garnish used here can be used for many other fish

4 x whole trouts, cleaned
30 ml (1 fl oz) olive oil
sea salt and freshly ground black pepper
120 g (4 oz) flaked almonds
juice of half a lemon
2 tbsp fresh tarragon leaves

■ Brush the trout with olive oil, season with salt and pepper and grill them until cooked — approx three minutes each side. Arrange the fish on serving dish and keep warm.

■ Heat remainder of olive oil in a clean frying pan until it starts to smoke, then add flaked almonds and toss rapidly over heat until golden brown.

■ Squeeze in lemon juice — it stops them colouring any more — remove from heat and pour mixture over the fish.

■ Sprinkle with the chopped tarragon and serve.

SCALLOPS IN TARRAGON CREAM

This recipe contains double cream, so be careful what else you plan on the same menu and use it for a special occasion, not an everyday meal.

| 1 tbsp olive oil spread |
| 700 g (1½ lb) fresh sea scallops |
| 2 tsp fresh tarragon leaves |
| sea salt and freshly ground black pepper |
| 60 ml (2 fl oz) double cream |
| 2 tbsp dry sherry (optional) |
| juice of 1 lemon |
| 1 tbsp chopped parsley |

■ Heat olive oil spread in large pan, on a fairly high heat, until it starts to foam.

■ Add the scallops and fresh tarragon, season with salt and pepper, and cook for two to three minutes stirring constantly.

■ Stir in double cream, dry sherry (if used) and lemon juice, turn down the heat and simmer until the scallops turn opaque and feel springy to the touch (this usually takes just a couple of minutes).

■ Remove the scallops and keep warm, reduce sauce until it is thick enough to coat the back of a wooden spoon, and stir in chopped parsley.

■ Arrange scallops on serving dish and coat with sauce. ▶

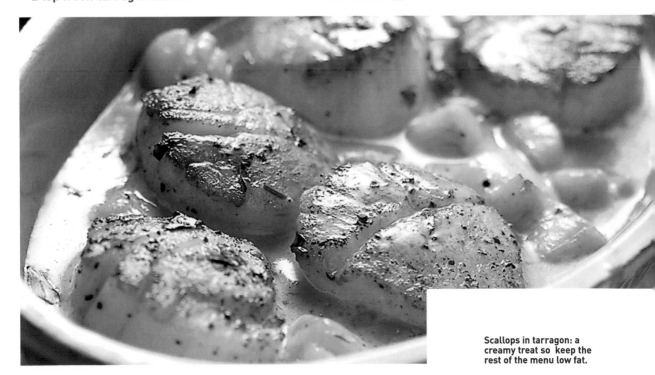

Scallops in tarragon: a creamy treat so keep the rest of the menu low fat.

POT ROAST CHICKEN

The perfect low maintenance Sunday lunch – put it on, spend three hours reading the papers then serve up ultra-tasty meat and vegetables!

2 large onions
1 leek
3 large carrots
2 celery sticks
a handful of button mushrooms
3 large cloves garlic
juice of 1 lime
freshly ground sea salt and black pepper
1.5 kg (3 lb) chicken (whole or jointed)
2 sprigs fresh parsley
2 spring fresh thyme
3 bay leaves

■ Rough cut the onion, leek, carrot and celery. Slice the mushrooms and garlic cloves and mix everything together.
■ Cover the inside of a lidded casserole dish with olive oil and pack the bottom with the chopped veg.
■ Wipe the lime juice over the chicken and season with salt and pepper.
■ Place chicken on bed of veg place parsley, thyme and bay leaves on top and cover with tight-fitting lid.
■ Bake in a medium oven for between 2—3 hours.
■ Discard sage, parsley and bay leaves, and serve chicken portions covered with veg and cooking juices.

Don't feel obliged to stop at chicken! Joints of beef, lamb and pork make fabulously tasty pot roasts, as the cooking method ensures no juices or flavour evaporate. Adjust the cooking times accordingly – a joint of beef of the same weight would take at least three hours, a joint of pork over four, and lamb somewhere in between.

NEXT DAY SOUP

If you prepare other vegetables to accompany the meat, the cooking juices, complete with pot roast veg can be cooled, stored in the fridge to be enjoyed the next day as a delicious soup. If there is not enough liquid when it is reheated, add chicken stock to make it up.

BROCCOLI & BACON QUICHE

The basic quiche filling recipe (cheese, eggs, milk and mustard) can be adapted to include other favourite ingredients, such as salmon and red peppers.

350 g (12 oz) olive oil tart crust dough (see page 148)
75 g (3 oz) back bacon
1 large head of broccoli
300 ml (½ pt) low-fat milk
2 eggs
75 g (3 oz) low-fat Cheddar cheese
1 tbsp finely grated parmesan cheese
2 tsp Dijon mustard (optional)
sea salt and freshly ground black pepper

■ Prepare dough as shown, line flan ring and put in fridge to relax.
■ Cut bacon across the rashers into strips and fry until cooked — it should show some browning.
■ Break off the broccoli florets and lightly steam, removing from heat before they are cooked all the way through — approximately two minutes.
■ In a large mixing bowl, combine milk, lightly beaten eggs, grated cheese, mustard and salt and pepper.
■ Carefully stir in bacon and broccoli florets and pour into relaxed but not cooked tart crust.
■ Bake in a moderate-to-hot oven for approximately 35 minutess. Test by inserting a knife into the centre; if it comes out clean, the filling is cooked. ▶

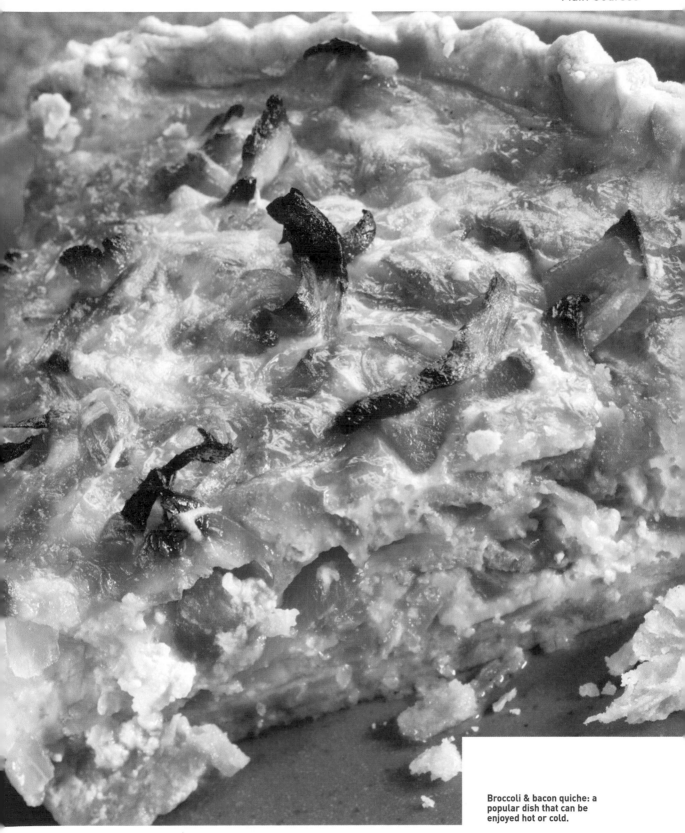

Broccoli & bacon quiche: a
popular dish that can be
enjoyed hot or cold.

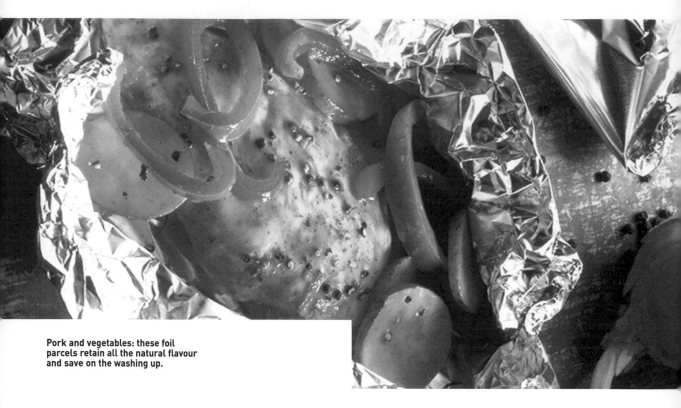

Pork and vegetables: these foil parcels retain all the natural flavour and save on the washing up.

STEAK SANDWICH WITH CARAMELIZED ONIONS

Such a substantial sandwich it is usually enough for a meal in itself.

2 large onions
2 tsp olive oil
120 ml (¼ pt) beef stock (one stock cube will make this)
½ tbsp brown sugar
1 tbsp balsamic vinegar
450 g (1 lb) thinly sliced frying steak
4 cloves garlic
sea salt and freshly ground black pepper
2 french loaves

To make the caramelized onions:
■ Slice the onions and fry in the oil until golden brown (approximately five minutes).

■ Add stock, brown sugar and vinegar to the pan, stir and boil rapidly until the liquid has reduced to a shiny glaze coating the onion slices.
To prepare the steaks:
■ Season the steaks with the chopped garlic, salt and plenty of black pepper and allow to stand for approx 10 minutes.
■ Fry in very hot oil, turning almost immediately, then removing just as quickly.
■ Slice the cooked steaks into strips and divide among the halved and split French loaves.
■ Top the steak with caramelized onions and put the top half on each sandwich.

Sliced button mushrooms or sliced red or green peppers are equally tasty candidates for caramelizing, and can be added to or substituted for the onion slices.

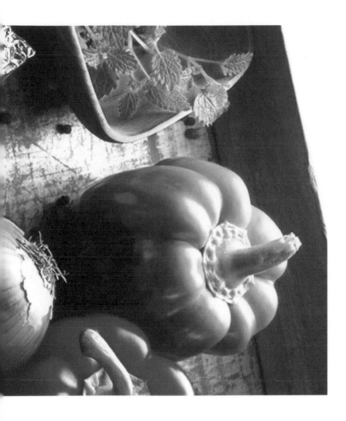

■ Combine orange juice, tomato purée, salt and pepper and parsley leaves.
■ Place each pork chop on the centre of a 30 x 45 cm (12 x 18 inch) piece of aluminium foil, cover with vegetables and drizzle with liquid.
■ Bring the long sides of each sheet of foil up to meet each other and double fold the edges to create an airtight seam all the way along.
■ Place in oven, seam upwards, and bake for approximately 30 minutes.
■ Serve in foil parcels opened at the table.

STEAK CHASSEUR
An example of classical French cuisine made healthy simply by leaving out the heavy sauce.

110 g (4 oz) button mushrooms
50 g (2 oz) shallots (button onions can be used as an alternative
2 cloves garlic
225 g (8 oz) fresh vine tomatoes
1 bunch fresh tarragon
sea salt
freshly ground black pepper
4 x sirloin steaks
60 ml (2 fl oz) white wine

■ Slice mushrooms and fry in olive oil, adding finely chopped shallots and garlic just before mushrooms are cooked.
■ Peel tomatoes, remove the pips and then dice flesh into squares.
■ Combine with roughly chopped tarragon leaves and add to mushrooms.
■ Season with salt and pepper.
■ Fry steaks.
■ Add white wine to the tomatoes and mushrooms and bring rapidly to the boil, allowing liquid to reduce slightly.
■ Arrange steaks on serving dish and cover with the sauce. ◻

EASY PORK AND VEGETABLES IN FOIL
Skinless chicken breasts can be used instead of pork if you prefer.

1 red pepper
1 green pepper
450 g (1 lb) small red potatoes
1 small onion
2 cloves garlic
1 tbsp orange juice
1 tbsp tomato purée
sea salt
freshly ground black pepper
1 tbsp flat parsley leaves
4 x boneless pork chops

■ De-seed and thinly slice peppers, potatoes and onions, finely chop garlic.

VEGETABLES

ALTHOUGH WE'VE ONLY INCLUDED A FEW RECIPES HERE, IT'S IMPORTANT TO EAT PLENTY OF VEGETABLES DAILY TO ENSURE A HEALTHY, BALANCED DIET. REMEMBER, STEAMED VEGETABLES RETAIN MORE FLAVOUR AND NUTRIENTS AND ARE LOW IN FAT.

SPANISH STYLE GREEN BEANS

These Mediterranean-style beans can be used as a hot vegetable dish or chilled down and served a salad.

450 g (1 lb) green beans
1 small green pepper
1 small red pepper
2 large cloves garlic
1 medium onion
1 large vine tomato
2 tbsp olive oil
sea salt and freshly ground black pepper
3 tbsp pitted black olives
2 tsp drained capers (optional)

■ Trim the green beans and cut them into 5 cm (2 in) lengths. Cut the green and red peppers into pieces roughly the same size as the green beans. Finely chop the garlic and chop onion into 1 cm (½ inch) squares. Peel the tomato, halve it, scoop out the seeds and cut flesh into pieces the same size as the onion.
■ Combine with the olive oil, salt and pepper, preheat a thick-bottomed pan on the stove and add vegetables.
■ Allow to sizzle for a couple of minutes, turn heat down, cover and cook until beans are just turning tender (approx 10–12 minutes).
■ Add chopped olives and capers (if using), cook for a further minute – just until olives are warmed through – and serve.

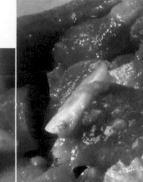
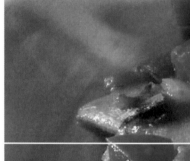
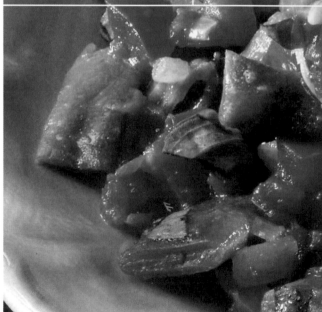

Roast mixed vegetables: the perfect side dish for your Sunday roast.

ROASTED MIXED VEGETABLES

The ideal accompaniment to roast meat as they can be cooked in the oven at the same time.

4 large carrots
4 medium potatoes
2 red peppers
2 green peppers
1 bulb garlic

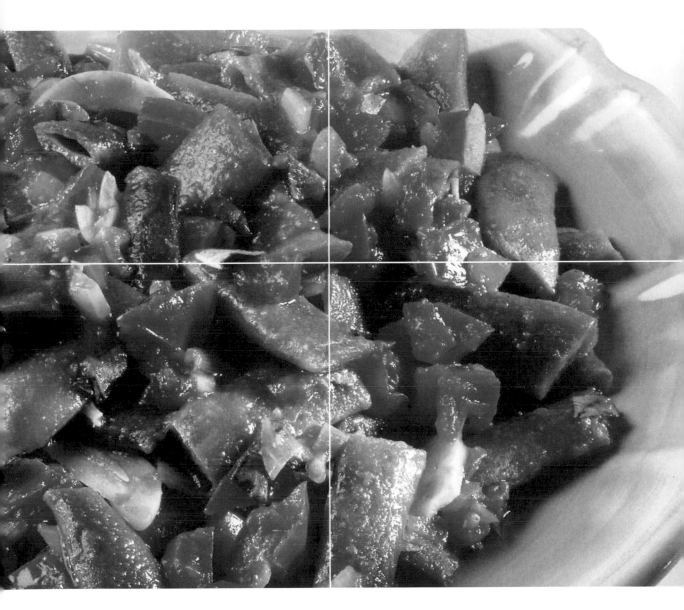

4 small onions

sea salt and freshly ground black pepper

2 tbsp olive oil

1 lime

1 tbsp of chopped, fresh flat parsley

■ Peel carrots and cut into large pieces — 2.5 cm (1 in) long, and halved or quartered — and, leaving the skin on, cut potatoes into large pieces. Steam

potato and carrot pieces until partially cooked.

■ De-seed and cut peppers into large pieces, peel garlic cloves and onions.

■ Put all the vegetables — steamed and raw — into a bowl, season and mix with olive oil and lime juice and parsley. Cover and leave overnight.

■ Place the vegetables and marinade on baking sheet and bake in a hot oven, turning frequently until golden brown — approximately 20 minutes. ▶

SNACKS & DRINKS

THE KIDS WILL LOVE THESE IN THEIR PACKED LUNCHES OR AS AFTER-SCHOOL TREATS.

PEANUT BUTTER SHAKE
Popular with children of all ages

300 ml (½ pt) low-fat milk
2 tbsp smooth peanut butter
1 small ripe banana
2 tbsp wheat germ

■ Toast the wheat germ and set a small amount aside.
■ Combine milk, peanut butter, banana and a large part of the wheat germ in a blender and mix until smooth and creamy.
■ Pour into glass and sprinkle the remainder of the wheat germ on top.

BERRY BERRY SMOOTHIE
The perfect long cool summer drink – and a dash of vodka or tequila can totally transform it into a sophisticated cocktail.

110 g (4 oz) frozen fresh raspberries
110 g (4 oz) frozen fresh strawberries
150 ml (5 fl oz) fresh pineapple juice
240 ml (8 fl oz) low-fat milk

■ Place fruit and fruit juice in blender and purée. Gradually add milk, blending until smooth before adding more.

The strawberries and raspberries can be substituted for the same amounts of fruit such as peaches, pears, blueberries, blackberries, bilberries and apricots. Avoid citrus fruit in case it curdles the milk. ▶

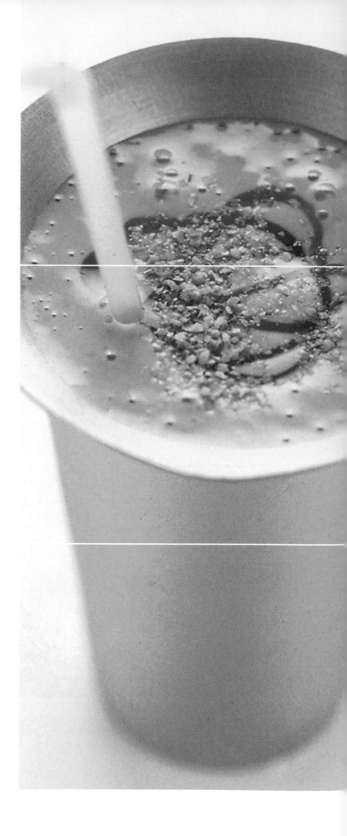

Peanut butter shake: a thick and nutritious drink.

Berry berry smoothie: cool and refreshing.

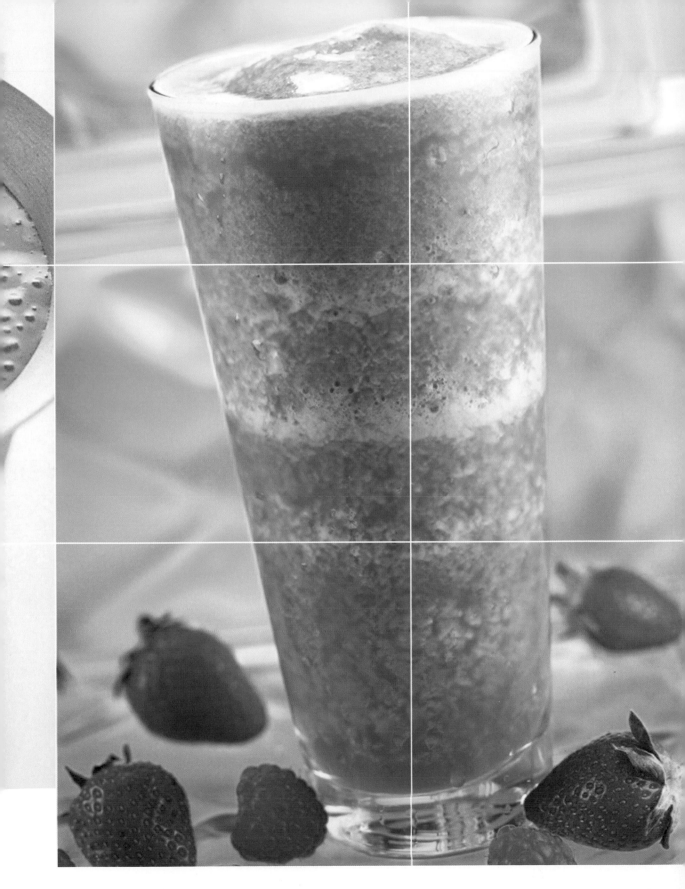

ITALIAN SALSA AND DIPPERS

These are ideal snacks to serve with drinks or to dig into while watching TV. Share with friends and family.

SALSA

5 plum tomatoes
1 small onion
3 cloves garlic
2 tbsp pitted black olives
2 tbsp fresh basil leaves
1 tbsp olive oil
3 tbsp balsamic vinegar
sea salt and freshly ground black pepper

■ Peel and chop the tomatoes – insides as well as the flesh – into 1 cm (½ in) squares. Finely chop onion, garlic, olives and basil leaves.
■ Combine in a bowl with oil, vinegar, salt and pepper and serve.

DIPPERS

4 pitta breads
25 g (1 oz) parmesan cheese
1 tsp paprika powder
1 tbsp finely chopped parsley

■ Cut pittas into wedge shapes and split.
■ Place on baking sheet and brush with olive oil.

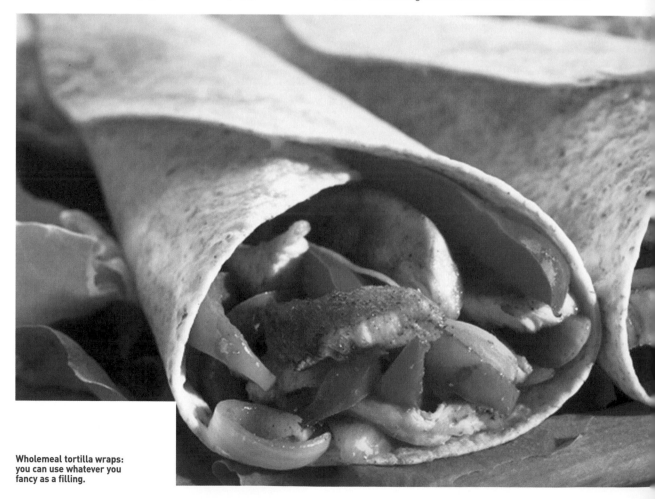

Wholemeal tortilla wraps: you can use whatever you fancy as a filling.

■ Combine parmesan, paprika and parsley and sprinkle liberally over pittas.
■ Bake in a hot oven until crisp and serve on a platter next to bowls of salsa dip.

WHOLEMEAL TORTILLAS
As versatile as sliced bread, but healthier!

560 g (1 lb 4 oz) wholemeal flour
1 tsp baking powder
pinch of sea salt
150 g (5 oz) olive oil spread
120 ml (4 fl oz) warm water

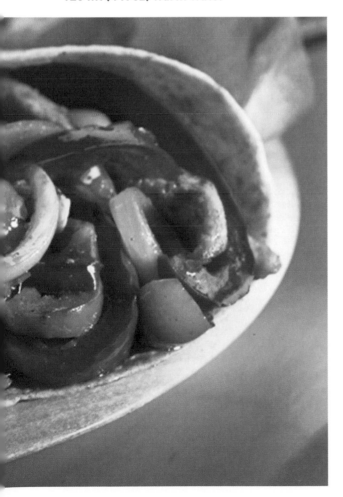

■ Sieve together flour, baking powder and salt in a large mixing bowl.
■ Cut the olive oil spread into cubes and rub into the flour. It should achieve a crumb-like consistency.
■ Gradually add the water, using enough to bring the mixture together into a stiff dough —you may need more than the 120 ml (4 fl oz).
■ Put dough on lightly floured surface and knead until elastic — about 15 minutes of working it into the table.
■ Divide dough into 12 even pieces and roll out each into discs approximately 30 cm (12 in) in diameter. To stop it from drying out, make sure to cover any dough not being worked on.
■ Fry each tortilla individually in a heavy pan on a medium heat for no more than a minute each side, until it starts to colour.
■ Keep cooked tortillas warm and soft by wrapping them in a clean tea towel.

Once you've made a dozen tortillas, there's an endless choice of fillings you can use. Here are a few ideas:

EGG AND BACON BURRITOS
Perfect for breakfast at the weekends

4 rashers bacon
6 eggs
sea salt
freshly ground black pepper

■ Remove the rind from bacon, fry and cut across into strips
■ Beat eggs, season with salt and pepper and add bacon strips.
■ Scramble in the usual way.
■ Divide among four warm tortillas, fold into classic burrito shape — put the filling in the middle, fold edges over to centre, then fold up ends into neat parcels — and serve. ▶

BEEF FAJITAS
Can be eaten cold as part of a packed lunch.

450 g (1 lb) thinly sliced frying steak
juice and zest of 2 limes
1 tbsp brown sugar
1 tsp chopped fresh oregano leaves
½ tsp cayenne pepper
2 cloves garlic
1 tsp ground cinnamon
2 small onions
1 red pepper
1 green pepper
1 yellow pepper
3 tbsp olive oil

■ Slice steak into 1 cm (½ in) strips, and combine in large mixing bowl with lime juice and zest, sugar, oregano, cayenne pepper, finely chopped garlic and cinnamon.

■ Marinade for at least an hour.

■ Slice onions and de-seeded peppers into 1 cm (½ in) strips.

■ Heat oil in large frying pan, add steak and marinade and fry for two minutes.

■ Add vegetable strips and continue cooking for another three minutes — veg should be cooked but still firm.

■ Spoon mixture on the centre of warm tortillas, roll up and serve.

CHICKEN SALAD ROLL-UPS
A family favourite for picnics.

3 oranges
2 spring onions
1 red pepper
6 iceberg lettuce leaves
½ cucumber
1 tbsp plum (or any seedless fruit) jam
1 tbsp balsamic vinegar
1 tsp fresh ginger root, grated
450 g (1 lb) cooked chicken breasts, shredded

■ Segment the oranges and drain slices, keeping back the juice.

■ Slice spring onions into 1 cm (½ in) slices, de-seed and cut pepper into 1 cm (½ in) squares, finely shred lettuce, de-seed and dice cucumber into 1 cm (½ in) pieces.

■ In a large mixing bowl combine jam, vinegar, orange juice and ginger into a sticky consistency — adjust quantities as necessary.

■ Add chicken and vegetables and mix well.

■ Spread on the middle of cold tortillas, roll up and serve.

CITRUS CRUSH
Probably the most refreshing drink you'll taste.

240 ml (8 fl oz) unsweetened pineapple juice
240 ml (8 fl oz) fresh orange juice
3 tbsp fresh lemon juice
2 tbsp fresh lime juice
a glass of crushed ice

■ Combine all ingredients in blender and puré e until smooth and frothy. Garnish with fruit slices.

ICED ORANGE-COCONUT DRINK
For an exotic twist use pineapple juice.

600 ml (1 pt) fresh orange juice
900 ml (1½ pt) unsweetened soya milk
300 g (10 fl oz) shredded coconut

■ Combine juice, milk and coconut in a blender and process until the mixture is smooth. Serve over ice in a tall glass. ◼

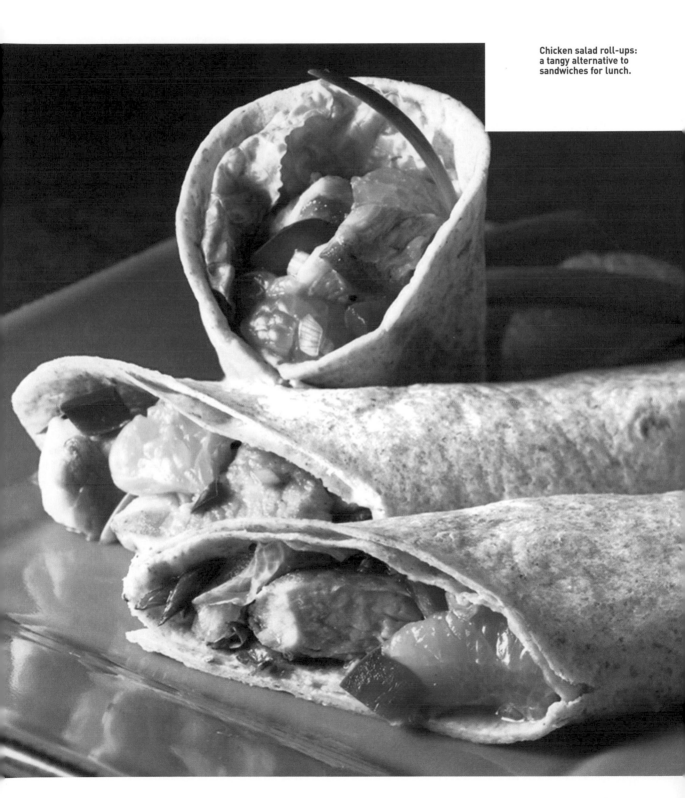

Chicken salad roll-ups: a tangy alternative to sandwiches for lunch.

CAKES & DESSERTS

NOW WE ARE AT THE GOOD BIT WHERE, WITH A FEW SIMPLE MODIFICATIONS, EVEN HEALTHY EATERS GET TO INDULGE THEIR SWEET TOOTH.

YOGHURT & MIXED FRUIT FLAN
The fruit suggested here for the topping can be substituted with your favourite fresh produce in season.

350 g (12 oz) tart crust dough (see page 150)
100 ml (3½ fl oz) low-fat natural yoghurt
1 dessertspoon runny honey
4 fresh peaches, peeled
2 kiwis, peeled
1 punnet raspberries
mint sprigs

■ Prepare dough as above, bake blind and leave to cool on wire rack.
■ Put yoghurt in a clean bowl and gradually add the honey, stopping before the mixture gets too sloppy. Spread over bottom of cooled crust.
■ Cut the peaches into thin wedges and the kiwis into slices, combine with the raspberries and arrange over the filling.
■ Drizzle any remaining honey across the arranged fruit and garnish with the sprig of mint.

BANANA BREAD
Can be eaten by itself or toasted with cinnamon butter.

110 g (4 oz) olive oil spread
225 g (8 oz) wholemeal flour
1 tsp bicarbonate of soda
2 eggs
2 large overripe bananas
2 tbsp low-fat milk ▶

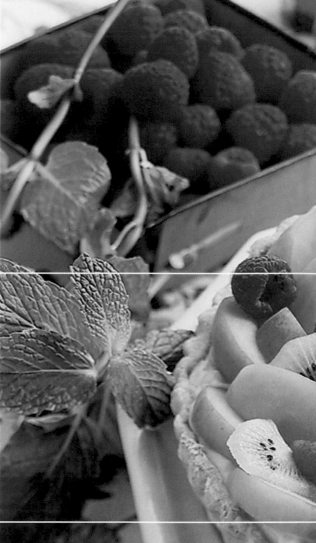

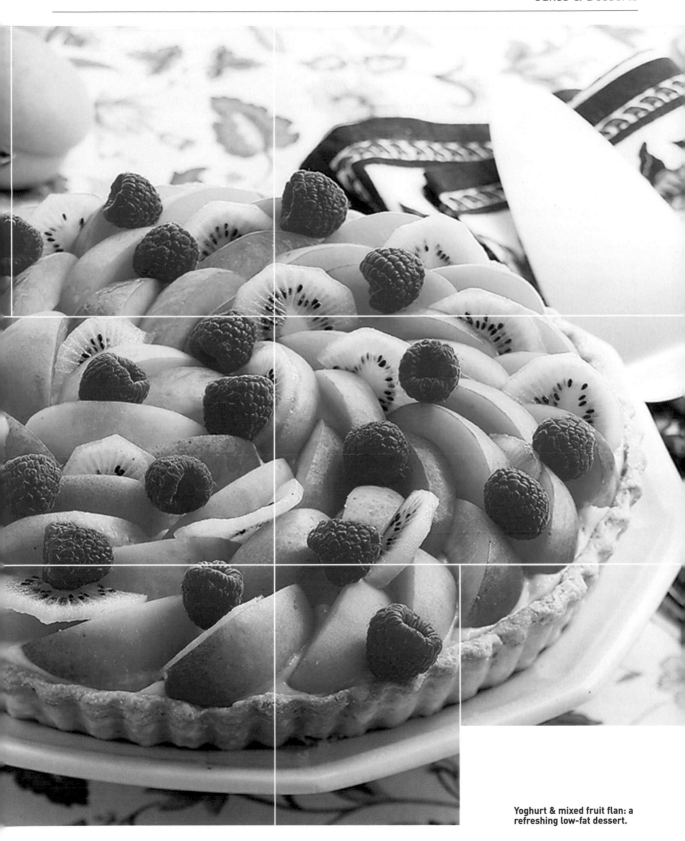

**Yoghurt & mixed fruit flan: a
refreshing low-fat dessert.**

■ Using an electric mixer, cream the olive oil spread until fluffy and nearly white.
■ Sieve the flour and bicarbonate of soda together and beat into the creamed olive oil spread.
■ Lightly beat the eggs in a separate bowl and gradually beat into the mixture.
■ Mash the bananas well – don't worry about discolouring – and stir into the mixture.
■ Gradually stir in the milk.
■ Pour into a greased loaf tin and bake at 180°C/350°F/ Gas mark 4 for 1-1¼ hours,
■ Turn on to a wire rack to cool.

OLIVE OIL TART CRUST
This delicious substitute for traditional pastry has endless possibilities for starters, main courses or desserts.

350 g (12o z) flour
1 tbsp caster sugar
½ tsp sea salt
5 tbsp olive oil
½ tsp white vinegar
2 tbsp water

■ Combine flour, sugar and salt in a large mixing bowl.
■ Stir in olive oil and vinegar until well combined.
■ Gradually mix in just enough water to hold it together as a firm dough.
■ Cover and put in the fridge to relax for at least 30 minutes.
■ Gently roll out and line a 30 cm (12 in) flan ring and put back in fridge for another 30 minutes.
■ To bake'blind', bake in hot oven (200°C/390°F/ Gas mark 6) until golden brown – approx 20 mins – remove and place on a wire rack to cool.

This versatile and delicious crust can be used with a number of different fillings or toppings, either sweet or savoury and served either hot or cold. A few examples follow, but feel free to let your imagination run away with you!

TARTE AUX POMMES
This adapts the classic French pastry to our healthy olive oil crust, but doesn't bake it blind as described left.

350 g (12 oz) tart crust dough (see left)
4 large dessert apples
1 tsp of brown sugar

■ Prepare dough as above, line flan ring and put in fridge to relax.
■ Peel, core and slice the apples and keep in a bowl of water until called for.
■ Dry apple slices on a clean tea towel, arrange in overlapping concentric circles on relaxed, uncooked tart crust.
■ Sprinkle with brown sugar.
■ Bake in hot oven (200°C/390°F/Gas mark 6) until golden brown – approximately 20 minutes. This tart can be left to cool on a wire rack, or served hot straight from the oven.

BASIC WHOLEMEAL CRÊPES
Use this recipe as the basis for lots of different desserts, changing ingredients accordingly

100 g (3 ½ oz) wholemeal flour
pinch sea salt
2 eggs
225 ml (8 fl oz) low-fat milk
1 dessertspoon of butter, melted
butter for frying

■ Sieve the all the flour and salt together into a large mixing bowl.
■ Using a wooden spoon, make a well in the centre of the flour.

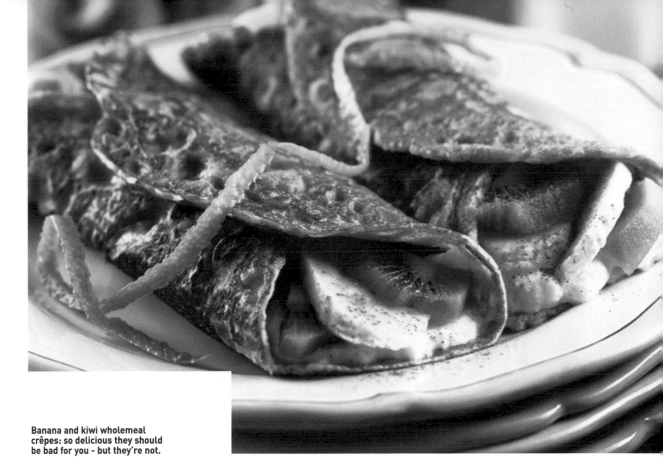

Banana and kiwi wholemeal crêpes: so delicious they should be bad for you – but they're not.

■ In a separate bowl, lightly beat the eggs and milk together.

■ Pour mixture carefully into the well in the flour and salt.

■ Using a whisk gradually incorporate the flour into the liquid and whisk to a smooth batter.

■ If there are a noticeable amount of lumps, pass through sieve into a jug or clean bowl.

■ Put the batter mix in the fridge to rest for at least half an hour.

■ Heat a knob of butter in a small frying pan until it starts to smoke. If the butter gets so hot as to turn black, it is burnt and will taint the taste of anything cooked in it.

■ Remove the pan from the heat, pour the butter away and wipe the pan out thoroughly with dry kitchen paper. Do not get the inside of the pan wet or the crêpes will stick.

■ Pour in a ladleful of batter and tilt the pan until it coats the base thinly – you should almost be able to see through the batter.

■ Fry quickly until crêpe appears to be set on top, turn it over – only attempt to toss it if,

a) you know what you're doing; or b) aren't very hungry! – and cook the other side for approximately 30 seconds.

■ Transfer to a plate with the first side to be cooked face down, and repeat cooking process with another ladle of batter.

■ Stack the cooked crêpes on top of each other so they don't dry out before serving.

BUCKWHEAT CRÊPES
Substitute half of the wholemeal flour for buckwheat flour and proceed as above

BANANA & KIWI CRÊPES
How can something this tasty be so healthy? Use a stack of warm crêpes, prepared from the basic crêpe mix shown left

2 bananas cut into slices
4 kiwi, peeled and sliced
juice of 1 lime
100ml (3½fl oz) natural set yoghurt
powdered cinnamon ▶

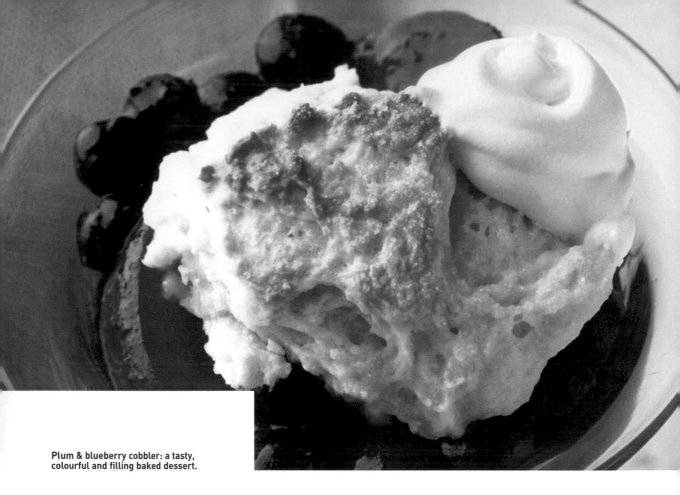

Plum & blueberry cobbler: a tasty, colourful and filling baked dessert.

■ Combine banana and kiwi slices in a bowl and sprinkle with lime juice.

■ Taking a crêpe from the stack, place evenly browned side down (that's why they should be stacked with the other, less attractive side upwards, so they don't have to be turned over again), and spread with a tablespoon of yoghurt, stopping just short of the edge.

■ Arrange a banana, a generous spoonful of kiwi and a banana in a strip across the crêpe, approximately two-thirds of the way from one edge.

■ Sprinkle with a pinch of cinnamon.

■ Gently roll up the crêpe, from the edge nearest the strip of filling.

■ Repeat for the remainder of the crêpes.

STRAWBERRY CRÊPES

Treat yourself to a taste of luxury. These creamy strawberry pancakes are a little bit naughty – but very nice!

50 g (2 oz) low-fat, cream cheese
150 ml (¼ pt) low-fat sour cream
a few drops vanilla essence
grated zest of 1 lemon
3 punnets fresh strawberries
1 tsp of caster sugar
squeeze of lemon juice

■ With a wooden spoon, in a large mixing bowl, beat together cream cheese, sour cream, vanilla and lemon zest until blended smooth.

■ Wash the strawberries and slice up two punnets' worth.

■ Taking a crêpe from the stack, with evenly browned side down, spread mixture over the surface, stopping just short of the edge.

■ Liberally sprinkle with strawberry slices, carefully fold each crêpe in half, then in half again.

■ In a food processor, purée the remainder of the strawberries with the sugar and a squeeze of lemon juice, to a rough, shiny sauce.

■ Arrange the folded crêpes on a serving dish and drizzle with sauce.

SOFT FRUIT CRÊPES

Any soft fruit can be used as a delicious filling for these crêpes. Take a small amount of the fruits and make into a purée (see method left) – this will bind the fruit together allowing it to spread on the crêpe.

PLUM & BLUEBERRY COBBLER

This baked dessert is surprisingly filling so a little goes a long way. If you can't get plums, try peaches or apricots instead.

8 fresh plums, quartered
225 g (½ lb) fresh blueberries
110 g (4 oz) brown sugar
175 g (6 oz) wholemeal flour
pinch sea salt
1 tsp baking powder
30 ml (1 fl oz) olive oil
120 ml (4 fl oz) low-fat buttermilk

■ In a large mixing bowl combine plums, blueberries, half of the sugar and two tablespoons of flour, and pour into greased baking dish.

■ In a medium mixing bowl combine remaining flour, sugar, salt and baking powder.

■ In another bowl, mix oil and buttermilk together, then add to the flour, mixing into a stiff batter.

■ Spoon the batter into individual 'islands' on top of the fruit.

■ Sprinkle with brown sugar and bake in a hot oven for 35–40 minutes until golden brown.

■ Garnish with a blob of low-fat fromage frais.

CORNMEAL FLAPJACKS

A breakfast favourite, the ideal substitute for toast.

225 g (8 oz) cornmeal
175 g (6 oz) wholemeal flour
1 tsp baking powder
1 egg
½ tsp sea salt
300 ml (½ pt) low-fat buttermilk
2 tbsp maple syrup
1 tbsp vegetable oil

■ In a large mixing bowl sieve together the cornmeal, flour, baking powder and salt.

■ In another bowl lightly whisk the buttermilk, egg, maple syrup and oil until fully blended.

■ Gradually add the liquid to the flour mix, beating it into a smooth batter. Sieve out any lumps and leave to rest for 20 minutes or so.

■ Heat a large, preferably thick-bottomed frying pan and lightly oil. Pour the batter in a ladleful at a time, keeping each flapjack separate

■ On a medium heat, cook for two minutes, until tiny bubbles appear on the surface and the edges begin to look dry. Flip and cook the other side for a minute or so.

■ Serve topped with fresh fruit or a drizzle of maple syrup.

OAT FLAPJACKS

If you don't eat all of these for breakfast, you can try them cold as cookies or to accompany a selection of cheeses.

150 g (5 oz) wholemeal flour
50 g (2 oz) porridge oats
1 tsp baking powder
½ tsp sea salt
25 g (1 oz) brown sugar
1 egg   ▶

1 tbsp vegetable oil

300 ml (½ pt) low-fat milk

Prepare as for cornmeal flapjacks, combining the dry ingredients in a large mixing bowl, then adding the prepared liquid to form a batter. Fry and serve using the same methods too. As a serving tip, these oatmeal flapjacks lend themselves better to savoury toppings or a part of a traditional breakfast.

BAKED LEMON RICE PUDDING
Limes or oranges are just as tasty, or add a handful of raisins.

50 g (2 oz) pudding rice (short grain)

40 g (1½ oz) caster sugar

grated zest of 2 lemons

600 ml (1 pt) low-fat milk

15 g (½ oz) butter

■ Wash rice and put in earthenware pie dish.
■ Add sugar, lemon zest and milk and mix well.
■ Dot with butter, place on baking sheet, and bake until the milk begins to boil.
■ Turn down heat and cook until a golden brown skin has formed – at least 90 minutes.

CANTALOUPE SORBET
A sophisticated dinner party dessert, that is equally good for the kids!

2 large cantaloupe melons

1 banana

1 tbsp caster sugar

1 tbsp crème de menthe (or whatever your favourite liqueur is)

1 lime

a pinch of ground cinnamon

fresh mint

■ Halve melons and carefully scoop out flesh, keeping half rinds intact.
■ Roughly chop and freeze flesh until still slightly soft to touch, not solid.
■ Slice and freeze banana.
■ Put the frozen fruit, all other ingredients and the juice and zest of the lime in a food processor and purée.
■ Freeze in a shallow pan, then break frozen mixture into chunks and lightly process into a smooth frozen slush.
■ Arrange in scooped-out shells and serve garnished with sprigs of fresh mint.

MUFFINS
A basic wholemeal muffin mix.

350 g (12 oz) wholemeal flour

2 tsp baking powder

1 tsp baking soda

pinch of sea salt

50 g (2 oz) brown sugar

200 ml (7 fl oz) low-fat buttermilk

60 ml (2 fl oz) olive oil

1 egg

grated zest of 1 lemon

■ Into a medium bowl sieve together flour, baking powder and soda and salt.
■ Keep back a teaspoonful of the sugar, and in a large mixing bowl combine the rest of it with the buttermilk, oil, egg and lemon zest until well blended.
■ Stir in flour until just combined – never beat, and take care not to overmix, as it doesn't matter if the muffin batter is lumpy.
■ Oil the bottom only of each compartment of a 12-muffin tin.
■ Fill two-thirds of the tin with batter and sprinkle the top of each with a pinch of sugar, for a crunchy textured top.

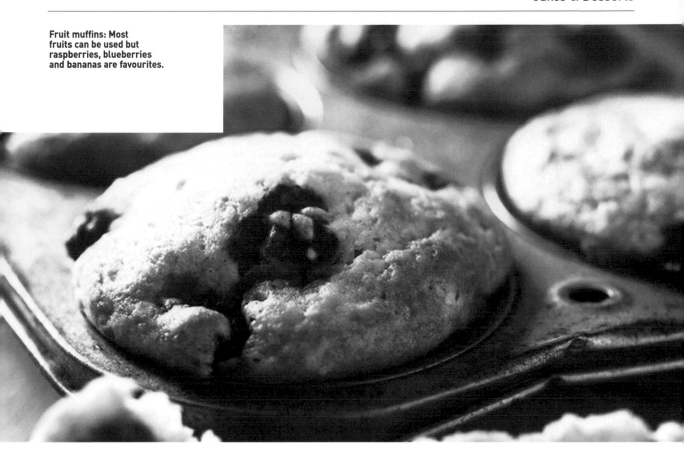

Fruit muffins: Most fruits can be used but raspberries, blueberries and bananas are favourites.

■ Bake in a preheated oven (200°C/390°F/ Gas mark 6) until risen and golden brown (approximately 15 minutes).

Although plain baked muffins like this can be a good substitute for bread, this basic batter can also be used for a seemingly infinite number of varieties of muffin.

APPLE MUFFINS
Fill each muffin tin with half the usual amount of batter, add a quarter of peeled and cored apple to each, top off with the remainder of the batter and bake as above. These will come out of the oven looking like ordinary muffins but when broken into will reveal the apple surprise.

FRUIT MUFFINS
This basic muffin mix will support about 200 g (7 oz) of fruit, which should be gently folded in to the batter just before it is poured into the tins.

Raspberries, strawberries, blueberries, peaches, apricots, dates or bananas are particular favourites, with the fruit being chopped as appropriate. If the fruit is particularly wet, like raspberries, cut back slightly on the liquid content of the batter.

NUT MUFFINS
Adding chopped walnuts, pecans or peanuts to the batter provides a wonderful crunchy texture as well as a great taste. About 110 g (4 oz) of chopped nuts is ideal for the above mixture, but remember to reduce the flour content by about 50 g (2 oz), otherwise they will come out too dry.

YOGHURT MUFFINS
For a fabulously unexpected taste, substitute equal amounts of yoghurt for buttermilk and, as it is heavier, add an extra half teaspoon of baking powder. These muffins can be especially tasty if you use fruit yoghurt. ◻

DIABETES DIRECTORY

KNOWLEDGE IS POWER IN THE BATTLE AGAINST DIABETES. FIND ALL
THE INFORMATION YOU NEED TO KNOW ON THESE WEBSITES.

DIABETES ORGANIZATIONS

Children with Diabetes
www.childrenwithdiabetes.com

Diabetics and diabetes
www.diabetes-and-diabetics.com

Diabetes Exercise and Sports Association
www.diabetes-exercise.org

Diabetes Health Online
www.diabetes.healthcentersonline.com

Diabetes Insight
www.diabetes-insight.info

Diabetes Mall
www.diabetesnet.com

Diabetes Network International
www.dni.org.uk

Diabetes Scotland
www.diabetes-scotland.org

The Diabetes Travel Information Website
www.diabetes-travel.co.uk

Diabetes UK
www.diabetes.org.uk

Insulin Pumpers UK
www.insulin-pumpers.org.uk

International Diabetes Federation
www.idf.org

Juvenile Diabetes Research Foundation
www.jdrf.org.uk

National Institute of Diabetes & Digestive & Kidney Diseases
www.niddk.nih.gov

ALTERNATIVE AND COMPLEMENTARY THERAPIES

Ayurveda
www.ayurveda.uk.com

British Acupuncture Council
www.acupuncture.org.uk

British Complementary Medicine Assoc
www.bcma.co.uk

The British Herbal Medicine Association
www.ex.ac.uk

British Homeopathic Association
www.trusthomeopathy.org

British Medical Acupuncture Association
www.medical-acupuncture.co.uk

The British Wheel of Yoga
www.bwy.org.uk

Tai Chi Union
www.taichiunion.com

Transcendental Meditation
www.t-m.org.uk/

The Qigong Centre
www.qimagazine.com

SUBJECT INDEX

RECIPE INDEX